D0090430

AN EMPOWERING GUIDE TO LUNG CANCER

AN EMPOWERING GUIDE TO LUNG CANCER

Six Steps to Taking Charge of
Your Care and Your Life

ERIC PRESSER, MD

Foreword by Andrew Ordon, MD

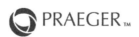 PRAEGER™

An Imprint of ABC-CLIO, LLC
Santa Barbara, California • Denver, Colorado

Library of Congress Cataloging-in-Publication Data

Names: Presser, Eric, author.
Title: An empowering guide to lung cancer : six steps to taking charge of your
   care and your life / Eric Presser, MD; foreword by Andrew Ordon, MD.
Description: Santa Barbara, California : Praeger, An Imprint of ABC-CLIO,
   LLC, [2017] | Includes bibliographical references and index.
Identifiers: LCCN 2016029949 (print) | LCCN 2016030916 (ebook) |
   ISBN 9781440841019 (alk. paper) | ISBN 9781440841026 (ebook)
Subjects: LCSH: Lungs—Cancer. | Lungs—Cancer—Diagnosis. |
   Lungs—Cancer—Treatment.
Classification: LCC RC280.L8 P74 2017 (print) | LCC RC280.L8 (ebook) |
   DDC 616.99/424—dc23
LC record available at https://lccn.loc.gov/2016029949

ISBN: 978-1-4408-4101-9
EISBN: 978-1-4408-4102-6

21 20 19 18 17   1 2 3 4 5

This book is also available as an eBook.

Praeger
An Imprint of ABC-CLIO, LLC

ABC-CLIO, LLC
130 Cremona Drive, P.O. Box 1911
Santa Barbara, California 93116-1911
www.abc-clio.com

This book is printed on acid-free paper ∞
Manufactured in the United States of America

Contents

Step VI. Acceptance

Foreword

In the popular press, I'm sometimes referred to as "America's Plastic Surgeon." However, what many people don't realize is that I'm also a board-certified otolaryngologist, specializing in head and neck surgery. As such, I've treated a number of cancer patients. I remember one woman who came to see me with a nagging cough she couldn't shake. It's not unusual for such a patient to seek out an ear, nose, and throat specialist (ENT). Many common ailments ENTs treat, including acid reflux, allergies, and postnasal drip, can trigger a persistent cough. After a suspicious-looking spot turned up on her chest X-ray, however, I began to suspect that cancer could be at the root of my patient's cough. Fortunately, we have tests today to screen for lung cancer at its earliest stages, before symptoms appear.

Patients with head and neck cancer frequently develop a second primary lung tumor, typically from smoking. We've all seen patients with head and neck cancers who develop a lung mass, the treatment of which depends on whether we're seeing a new metastasis or new primary lung cancer. We're fortunate that the advent of minimally invasive technology has allowed us to make a definitive diagnosis with less pain, scarring, and hospitalization.

I've always had a special affinity for cancer patients. Those whom I've had the privilege of knowing and treating have a life perspective that has enriched and challenged me as a physician and as a person. I feel humbled and stand in bewildered awe of the many cancer patients and their families who have allowed me to experience some of the most intimate details of their lives. Although a cancer diagnosis is a devastating blow even for the hardiest of souls, I have witnessed that this bad news can also produce the opposite effect, bringing out the best in my patients and their loved ones.

It's for these reasons that I'm thrilled to write the foreword for my friend and colleague Dr. Eric Presser's powerful new book, AN EMPOWERING GUIDE TO LUNG CANCER. This book is for anyone whose life has been touched by lung cancer and is looking for more effective strategies for preventing and treating this life-altering illness and the suffering it causes. As physicians, it's critical we offer patients encouragement, as well as treatment. Thus, I am always on the lookout for tools that will help them navigate through difficult issues that inevitably arise. AN EMPOWERING GUIDE TO LUNG CANCER is one such tool. Dr. Presser's book is something that I could offer not only to my patients and their families, but also to my own family, colleagues, and friends. It's not a book with all the answers (there is no such book), but it is a solid foundation for constructing an understanding of what's needed to deal with lung cancer.

Why do I say that I want to give this book to my family, colleagues, and friends rather than just my patients and their loved ones? The reason is simple: Because virtually everyone I know will be affected in some way by lung cancer. This is not particularly surprising, as lung cancer is the leading of cause of cancer death worldwide and the leading cancer killer of men and women in the United States, claiming more lives than colorectal, breast, and prostate combined. Although lung cancer takes more than a million lives annually, there are a significant number who survive as well. The American Lung Association reports that the five-year survival rate for lung cancer is 54 percent for cases detected when the disease is still localized. Yet only 15 percent of lung cancer cases are diagnosed at Stage I, buttressing the need for early diagnosis and prevention.[1] The bottom line: As we thankfully grow older and hopefully live longer, lung cancer will touch each of our lives in some way.

Aristotelian principles have long guided and governed the practice of medicine, the idea being that an understanding of the disease precedes experimentation and treatment. This isn't an unreasonable approach; responsible doctors should try to understand the nature of the ailment they're addressing and then consider an intervention—be it an operation, medication, or a psychiatric therapy—that goes to the root the problem. And this method works, most of the time. It's based on a simple, rational premise: Know the problem, and the solution will reveal itself.

But even the most skilled and experienced physician can't know everything. Cancer is a tricky illness. Its cells adroitly mount defenses against the treatments we develop. A lung cancer patient may receive a targeted therapy that reduces or eliminates a tumor, only to have the cancer return a short time later. Cancer is a varied, multisystem disease, and its treatments are multimodal. A lung cancer patient may undergo one, two, or even multiple treatments, including surgery, chemotherapy, radiation, targeted drug therapy, hormone therapy, and biotherapy. Cancer treatments may last for months, if not years, each having a radically different effect on a person's quality of life. Eric Presser is a specialist in minimally invasive lung cancer surgery and a recognized expert on the benefits of early detection through low-dose CT (computed tomographic) screening. But lung cancer isn't a solo affair; treatment is a coordinated effort, involving oncologists, radiologists, surgeons, and geneticists, among many others. Moreover, lung cancer patients have quality-of-life concerns that involve physical, psychological, and practical issues. Improvements in treatments and early diagnosis have extended the survival rates for lung cancer patients. Like all cancer patients, lung cancer patients have unique health and support needs. Lung cancer, as with most cancers, is a disease of aging. Although there is a commonality of experiences among patients who have undergone lung cancer treatment, the elderly have quality-of-life concerns that differ from the rest of the population. Similarly, many lung cancer patients, who crave control over their illness and want to do everything possible to restore their health, seek out complementary and alternative therapies.

What impressed me so much about the approach offered in AN EMPOWERING GUIDE TO LUNG CANCER is Eric Presser's willingness to look to outside sources for those things that fall outside his area of expertise. His extensive consultations with experts, including physicians, mental health professionals, and folks working in the field of complementary and alternative medicine, have added a layer of credibility to the information presented here. No physician or medical society is going to agree with or vouch for every page of this book. Achieving that level of consensus is impossible, and I'd add not even desirable. Treating a disease like lung cancer requires an ability to think outside the box.

AN EMPOWERING GUIDE TO LUNG CANCER is a book that I want to have and want others to have. Professional organizations such as the American Cancer Society, the American Association for Cancer

Research, and American Society for Clinical Oncology provide terrific up-to-date information on a variety of cancer topics but can't possibly offer the anecdotal, day-to-day, how-to-live-with-lung-cancer information in this book.

It's unfortunate that many people who come face-to-face with the need to understand lung cancer are overwhelmed by the myriad available Internet resources, as well as the usual misinformed advice from well-meaning friends, neighbors, and even some health care professionals. Although all of the factual information in this book is attainable through other means, I haven't encountered another book on lung cancer that provides this kind of comprehensive format with information and wise guidance framed in a reassuring manner.

The book is not just about lung cancer. It's also about problem solving, about living and thriving, about finding meaning and hope even when faced with difficult circumstances, and about striving to live as long and as well as possible. AN EMPOWERING GUIDE TO LUNG CANCER will inspire as well as inform you. What could be better than that?

Andrew Ordon, MD

Preface

Mary's Story

"But I never smoked, maybe a cigarette here or there in college, but that's all. Lung cancer happens to smokers. Doesn't it?"

After a decade as a practicing thoracic surgeon specializing in lung cancer, I have had those words thoroughly drummed into my consciousness. This time, they were coming from the mouth of Mary, a 60-years-young dancer and fitness fanatic. The image of the archetypal lung cancer patient is etched into our collective awareness: the stained yellow teeth and fingers, the prematurely aged eyes framed in dark circles, the shriveled lips, and the desiccated, brittle hair.

This wasn't Mary. The woman standing in front of me had soft hazel eyes gleaming with exuberance; her long, flowing auburn hair flecked with gunmetal gray streaks. Pristine porcelain skin covered a handsome, alert face that tapered into beautiful red lips and an angelic smile.

The other thing about cancer is that it happens to the proverbial "other person," the one exposed to a toxic cocktail of smoking and drinking. You know, the fat guy or gal who doesn't exercise or spends his or her day in a hazardous work environment, bombarded constantly by a smorgasbord of mysterious carcinogens. Mary's unrelenting cough and hoarseness were probably just remnants of a determined cold, or at worst bronchitis, a condition easily treated with antibiotics.

In fact, it was a persistent cough that brought Mary into my hospital. Just a week earlier, she'd been playing hide-and-go-seek, as she often did, with her five young grandchildren. But something felt different this time. Within minutes, Mary was hunched over and out of breath, so much so that she was forced to stop playing and sit down. Not wanting to disappoint her grandkids, who always looked forward to spending time with her, Mary quickly regained her composure and returned to the game. Still, she couldn't shake the nagging sense that something was terribly wrong. Over the past six months, there were a number of occasions when she'd found herself out of breath for no apparent reason.

The persistent cough was of greatest concern to Mary. She'd always been active, even after retiring from her job as co-artistic director of a regional ballet company. Daily walks with her husband, tennis, Pilates, and twice-weekly yoga classes were all part of this former professional dancer's regimen. Mary had always prided herself on being in pretty good shape.

One day, while out walking the dog, Mary couldn't catch her breath. Walking the family Pug wasn't typically a strenuous activity, so she felt somewhat alarmed to be in this predicament. "I felt like I was drowning," Mary told Paul when she got home. Paul drove her to the emergency room. After she underwent a full work-up, Mary was relieved to learn that she had not had a heart attack. The doctor also ordered a CT (computed tomography) scan to make sure she didn't have a blood clot in her pulmonary arteries, which could easily have contributed to her shortness of breath. Of concern to the doctors was what one of them described as an "excessive accumulation of fluid" in Mary's chest, which they detected during the scan. Before she could even blink, Mary was being asked to sign a consent form to have a needle stuck in her back. Draining fluid would allow the lung to re-expand. It all made sense to Mary. "Of course, get the fluid out. I want to go home," Mary replied immediately.

After the procedure to drain some of the fluid, known as a thoracentesis, the attending physician called me in for a consult. I greeted Mary in her hospital room on a cold, snowy Sunday afternoon. Mary's husband of 32 years, Paul, was there, sitting quietly, his eyes glued to the Giants–Eagles game. I'm a diehard Giants fan and would've liked nothing better than to pass the afternoon watching the game. But this was no time for frivolity, so I politely turned down the TV volume. The three of us needed to talk. I explained to Mary and Paul that additional fluid would have to be drained from her chest so her lung could re-expand and I could obtain a sample of tissue from inside her chest wall. This would give a definitive diagnosis because the results from the pleural fluid that had been drained from

Mary's lungs were suspicious but inconclusive. Mary's eyes glazed over as I explained the steps needed to help her breathe better and obtain a proper diagnosis. She was still in disbelief over the prospect that she might have lung cancer. "But I never smoked. Lung cancer happens to smokers," she kept repeating.

Mary was confused. Who wouldn't be under the circumstances? And she was scared, especially after she learned that I'd be cutting into her chest. Mary seemed relieved when she learned the "cut" would consist of nothing more than a one-centimeter incision, which would be used to drain the fluid that had accumulated between her lung and her chest wall. Through that same tiny incision, I'd also be able to biopsy the undersurface of Mary's chest wall, explore her chest cavity, and then decide the best way to keep her lungs expanded and help her breathe. With surgical patients, information—provided its presented in the right way—almost always allays fears and offers reassurance.

"Picture a blown-up balloon stuffed inside a two-liter soda bottle," I continued. "Think of the balloon as Mary's lung and the soda bottle as her chest cavity. If you pour any liquid into the bottle, the volume of the balloon will decrease because, in a closed space, the fluid always wins." I went on to explain that gluing the balloon to the sides of the soda bottle would result in the fluid having nowhere to accumulate. I explained to Mary and Paul that we needed to remove the accumulated fluid to see if the lung would expand completely. I would perform a pleurodesis, which is a procedure done to treat recurrent collapsed lungs or fluid buildup between the lung and chest wall lining that doesn't go away on its own. Pleurodesis helps optimize the lung's capacity to expand. The human body doesn't like empty spaces. A trapped lung or one that can't expand fully will fill the void with fluid. If this happened to Mary during the procedure, I could solve the problem by placing a small tube into her chest to help drain the fluid and keep the empty space dry. This would optimize her ability to expand the lung and also take pressure off the heart and other important structures in the chest. Draining fluid has an adjunctive benefit of taking pressure off the unaffected lung as well, allowing it to function optimally. Keeping the space dry gives the lung a chance to adhere to the chest wall, eliminating the space for the fluid to accumulate.

Mary and Paul seemed to grasp what I was saying, but her next question would prove more challenging. "What's my stage,

Dr. Presser?" I answered as gently as I could. "The fluid we drained from your lungs suggests Stage IV non–small cell lung cancer." Even a layperson knows that Stage IV is an advanced cancer benchmark.

Mary and Paul didn't have to say a word. Their faces told me all I needed to know. As I talked, I could feel Paul drifting away, his attention slowly returning to the game, a welcome distraction from the nightmare I was laying at his feet. Mary took my hand and thanked me, her eyes welling with tears. I placed my hand over hers and looked into her eyes. "Thank me after you leave the hospital."

"What's your favorite type of music?" Mary seemed puzzled by my non-sequitur. "Don't answer now. Think about it and let me know tomorrow," I told her. I shook Paul's hand, turned the TV volume on, and made my way out of the room. The Eagles were down two touchdowns, but Paul looked relieved. I felt confident that Mary and Paul knew the first step, which was to help Mary breathe better. Coming up with a definitive diagnosis would be harder. But together with her oncologist, I knew we'd come up with a game plan.

The next morning, just before heading into the operating room, Mary and I reviewed her procedure one final time. Having never undergone surgery, Mary was afraid of being intubated, so I told her I would perform the procedure using only light sedation and a local anesthetic. This wouldn't adversely affect the results of the procedure and would bring Mary, who was already anxious, some peace of mind. I'd be performing an "awake" thoracoscopy or VATS (video-assisted thoracic surgery). I've been performing this procedure for years, and it works well for patients who cannot tolerate or are terrified of general anesthesia. Knowing that she wouldn't need to "go under" as she put it seemed to help Mary deal with the stress of surgery. Before surgery, the anesthesiologist administered the sedative Versed, which further helped Mary relax. Just as the anesthesia was starting to kick in, I heard Mary mumble "Johnny Cash." My colleagues looked puzzled; no one had any idea what she was talking about. I just smiled, walked over to my iPod, and put on "Ring of Fire."

During the procedure, I drained 1500cc of fluid and biopsied the tissue from Mary's chest wall. I could see her lung was trapped in many places from the cancer, preventing it from expanding fully. To help, I placed a small tube into Mary's chest cavity. At least she would be able to get out of the hospital in the morning. When Mary started to come to, I told her everything went as well as could be expected. She half-smiled, relieved but also saddened as she remembered her diagnosis of advanced lung cancer.

Two weeks later, Mary had already started chemotherapy. The pleural catheter I'd inserted was draining about 300 to 400cc of fluid every two days from in her chest. She looked healthy, and her spirits were high. Although her prognosis was poor (there was no getting around that reality) but at least she could breathe. The life expectancy of Stage IV lung cancer patients can vary considerably depending on such factors as the type and location of the cancer, age (younger people often live longer), sex (women with lung cancer live longer at each stage of lung cancer), general health at the time of diagnosis, response to treatment, co-occurring conditions, and complications of having advanced lung cancer. Many patients can tolerate pain, but there is something particularly vexing about not being able to breathe properly.

Mary returned to my office every month after the procedure. I removed the catheter after the fluid finished draining. The catheter had done its job, allowing the lung to stick up against the chest wall, preventing further fluid accumulation. "Mary, I know our work is done here, but feel free to call me if you need anything. Day or night, I'm just a phone call away." I reminded her that when it comes to lung cancer, statistics are just statistics and that everything is *treatable*, not necessarily *curable*, but everything is definitely *treatable*. "Thank you, Dr. Presser, for performing the procedure. But most of all, thank you for changing my outlook, doing away with my fear and giving me hope."

"Of course, and Mary, don't forget to show me a video of you playing with your grandchildren during our next visit."

When I have a case such as Mary's, I question whether there is any justice in the world. How does an otherwise healthy, vibrant, 60-year-old wife, mother, and grandmother contract Stage IV non–small cell lung cancer? Before her unexpected diagnosis, everything seemed *right* in Mary's world. But she had that damned cough that just wouldn't go away. Before receiving the diagnosis, I could tell that Mary knew something was wrong. But who's ever prepared to hear that they've got terminal cancer? I saw the look in both Mary's and Paul's eyes. No matter the outcome, they knew their lives had changed forever.

Going forward, Mary's life would be filled with many challenges. There would be joy, but also great sadness. As Mary's health slowly declined, there were periods when it seemed that all order had disappeared from her life. "She's the anchor. Nothing works without her," Paul confided to me after a particularly grueling chemotherapy session.

For more than a year after her death, nothing seemed right in Mary's family. But they're a resilient bunch. In time, they all crawled their way back to their lives, not surprisingly with, as Paul said, "a deeper sense of gratitude and renewed appreciation for each day." This was an enlightened perspective, particularly from a man who'd just lost his best friend and partner of 32 years.

My Mission

It's late, near the end of an excruciatingly long day that started at 5 AM with an emergency VATS (video-assisted thoracic surgery) to remove blood from the chest of a 21-year-old car accident victim who was rushed to the ER after suffering a hemothorax—the accumulation of blood in the space between the lung and chest wall. It's a serious, potentially life-threatening condition. Now, 15 hours later, I just want to go home. Unfortunately, I can't. Tonight is my hospital's "Autumn Benefit," a cocktail reception and dinner organized by a group called the Committee for Professional Medical Education. I'm beat. I can barely keep my eyes open. But this really is a worthwhile event, and the committee is truly dedicated to providing superior medical education and teaching the latest techniques in orthopedics, anesthesiology, cardiology, oncology, and, of course, thoracic surgery.

Just as I'm about to sit down to dinner, two women approach me. "So, what do you do?" one of them asks. It's loud, music is blaring, and there are a hundred separate conversations going on simultaneously. I lean in. "I'm a thoracic surgeon," I tell her. Immediately, her eyes light up. "Wow! You know, Doctor, I've been thinking of having my brow lifted and trying Botox. Then she points to her biceps. "I'm not happy with my arms either. Maybe I could use some liposuction. What do you think?" I smile. "No, I'm not a plastic surgeon. I'm a thoracic surgeon—I operate on chests." She looks slightly deflated. I feel badly for taking the wind out of her sails. "Of course, if I were smart, I'd be a plastic surgeon. Everyone likes to see them. No one likes to see me," I added, hoping to lighten the mood.

I hear them all the time and understand the sentiment. There's no open bar or free buffet in my office. My assistants don't hand out lollipops, balloons, or complimentary facial cream samples. I perform thoracic surgery, after all, the purpose of which is to treat diseases of and organs in the chest. And most of the diseases and conditions I treat—lung cancer, esophageal cancer, and pleural effusion—are just a few of the awful, life-threatening illnesses that I encounter.

But as recently as a decade ago, lack of knowledge was the most vexing aspect of dealing with lung cancer. Today, other questions are foremost on the mind of lung cancer patients. What's the best way to treat lung cancer? What if it can't be treated? Can lung cancer be prevented? Is surgery the answer? If not, what are the alternatives? AN EMPOWERING GUIDE TO LUNG CANCER isn't a book based on far-out principles, untenable cures, or magical thinking. It's decidedly not a triumph of serendipity over science and reason. Making life-changing decisions can only be done with proper, practical, and scientifically sound information. That's what AN EMPOWERING GUIDE TO LUNG CANCER offers. Anything less would be a disservice to you, the reader.

I can't take sole credit for the contents of this book. To write AN EMPOWERING GUIDE TO LUNG CANCER, I've drawn not only on my 17 years' experience as a physician specializing in minimally invasive lung cancer surgery, but on the expertise, experiences, and insight of colleagues, acquaintances, and friends whom I've grown to admire and trust. Most of all, I've come to rely most heavily on the experiences of my patients. They are my greatest teachers.

AN EMPOWERING GUIDE TO LUNG CANCER is written for anyone touched by this life-altering disease. It begins with two chapters that discuss the basics of the respiratory system (Chapter 1) and cancer (Chapter 2). The chapters that follow detail the six steps I recommend for taking charge of your care. Learning about lung cancer—its symptoms, causes, and treatment—will empower you to make sound, reason-based decisions and find the right solution. This book offers a major dose of prevention gospel, including ways to significantly minimize lung cancer risk through low-dose screening. I have no problem evangelizing when it comes to spreading the disease-prevention message. You'll learn how to plan for the future, the Achilles' heel for a significant percentage of late-stage cancer patients, surprisingly. Together, we'll figure out how you can have the best possible quality of life. With this book, you'll have the tools and resources to blaze a bold new path and make treatment decisions suited to your personality style and preferences.

As you might expect in a consumer-friendly health book, AN EMPOWERING GUIDE TO LUNG CANCER contains a number of medical terms. Don't freak out. Medical terminology is your friend. It's only intimidating because it's unfamiliar, like anything encountered for the first time. I didn't know a thoracotomy from a lobectomy when I started medical school. But don't forget that knowledge is power. It levels the playing field, bridging the often-tenuous doctor–patient communication gap.

AN EMPOWERING GUIDE TO LUNG CANCER is filled with anecdotes from the frontlines. I'm deeply indebted to my patients and their families—the people living with lung cancer—for sharing their unique and often painful circumstances and perspectives. In a world where we're conditioned to tap-dance around difficult subjects, I think you'll find their candor refreshing and relatable.

AN EMPOWERING GUIDE TO LUNG CANCER includes resources, dispersed throughout the text and at the end of this book, and "takeaways" at the beginning of each chapter to help you quickly and easily locate the resources you need. You can find additional resources on my personal website, www.anempowerguidetolung cancer.com.

While reading this book remember that because lung cancer is a complicated illness, there is no one-size-fits-all solution. Good treatment plans are highly individualized, taking into account the stage and/or disease manifestation, ancillary medical problems, personality type, and psychological well-being. Familial support and finances also factor in, although the latter should never be an issue, in my opinion. Seek advice from trusted medical professionals, but remember that even the most skilled and experienced physician isn't infallible. If you're uncomfortable with something you've been told, get a second opinion. This is your life.

"A good doctor never stops learning," said a professor on my first day of medical school. After devoting half my life to the study of medicine, I'd like to believe that I'm sufficiently immersed in and knowledgeable about the human body's most intimate details. But doctors don't know everything. As such, I solicited a number of colleagues to help write this book. All those asked willingly contributed their time, effort, and expertise. No one requested compensation. They shared my commitment to helping people living with lung cancer.

Most of all, AN EMPOWERING GUIDE TO LUNG CANCER is about helping people. It's a labor of love, nothing more. I didn't venture into this strange new world intent on writing a best seller—though that would be nice—or securing a lucrative publishing deal. In the final analysis, if you find that this book contributes in some small way to your well-being, then it's served its purpose.

The Basics

CHAPTER 1

The Respiratory System

Takeaways

- The human respiratory system consists of organs responsible for respiration, the process involved in taking in oxygen and expelling carbon dioxide. The lungs carry out the exchange of these two gases.
- The circulatory and respiratory systems are tag-team partners; working in tandem, they gather oxygen and transport it through the circulatory system. These systems also partner to eliminate carbon dioxide, a toxic, metabolic waste product. In humans, these two systems are connected in the lungs, the hub for the exchange of carbon dioxide and oxygen.
- Inhalation is the start of oxygen's path through the circulatory and respiratory systems. As you inhale, your diaphragm contracts, drawing air into the lungs. The air moves toward your lungs through a series of tubes that start from the nose and mouth. Once air reaches the lungs, it enters the alveoli, millions of small, specialized structures where the exchange of carbon dioxide and oxygen (CO_2 and O_2,) actually takes place.
- Red blood cells pick up oxygen in the lungs and carry it to every part of the human body.
- Every cell in your body requires oxygen to function properly.
- In humans, breathing rate depends on age. Newborns breathe 40 times per minute, slowing to 20 to 40 times per minute during sleep. The average resting respiratory rate for adults is 12 to 16 breaths per minute.

- The circulatory and respiratory systems meet at the alveoli and capillaries. As air makes contact with capillaries, oxygen diffuses through the capillary walls. Diffusion takes place because there is more oxygen in the lungs than in the surrounding blood. Oxygen molecules then enter the blood, where they bind to sites on red blood cells before dispersing throughout the body.

Introduction

Even if you failed high school biology or your science knowledge doesn't extend beyond a few episodes of the *Dr. Oz Show*, you probably know that your respiratory system helps you breathe. But why do we breathe? It's the process by which our bodies take in oxygen and expel carbon dioxide. It's a critical function because every human body needs oxygen and is adversely affected if that supply is impaired. An understanding of the respiratory system and its function offers a foundation for understanding how lung cancer affects the body.

Breathing

Breathing is the Big Kahuna, quite literally the human respiratory system's most essential function. With each inhalation, we fill our bodies with life-giving oxygen, which we can't do without for more than a few minutes. With each exhalation, we eliminate carbon dioxide, the gas produced by normal body processes. Lungs are the catalyst—the place for taking in oxygen and eliminating carbon dioxide.

Would you like to experience the body parts involved in breathing? Take a moment. Breathe in. Feel the air as it enters your nose or mouth. Notice as it passes quickly to the throat before being pulled down into the trachea, which branches into the right and left and bronchi. Before continuing with our discussion of air's path once it enters the lungs, let's consider the very act of breathing.

The diaphragm, a large, dome-shaped muscle that sits below the lungs and serves as the main muscle of respiration, separates the lungs and other chest organs from abdominal organs.[1] As we inhale, the diaphragm contracts and moves downward, increasing space in the chest cavity, which gives the lungs space to expand. A relaxed diaphragm, on the other hand, moves upward, pushing against the lungs, causing them to exhale. There are other muscles between the ribs that help facilitate the expanding and contracting cycle, but for our purposes, the diaphragm is the focus.[2]

Relaxed and Contented

Breathing is unique among bodily functions. What makes it so remarkable is that it's not simply an autonomic (involuntary) function. The autonomic nervous system (ANS), which controls breathing, has three wings or branches: the sympathetic nervous system (SNS—fight-or-flight response), the parasympathetic nervous system (PNS—rest and digest), and the enteric nervous system (regulates the gastrointestinal system). The PNS and SNS are tag-team partners, working in tandem, much like your car's gas pedal and brakes. Controlled breathing techniques can trigger these two branches, yielding a number of positive outcomes such as lowered stress, reduced blood pressure, and a fortified immune system. If you want to know what it's like to engage the ANS' parasympathetic branch, trying inhaling and exhaling deeply for 60 seconds (fill your lungs, hold for 1–2 seconds, and then exhale naturally).[3,4]

Controlled breathing can be therapeutic for lung cancer patients, many of whom live with the specter of a disease course and treatment that seems beyond their influence and control. Meditation, yoga, balancing heart rate variability, specific nostril breathing (known as *pranayama*), body mindfulness, yawning, and increasing positive emotion are among a handful of scientifically proven techniques that can help activate the PNS and SNS.[5] A number of Eastern spiritual traditions, including yoga and tai chi, make great use of controlled breath work.[6]

Breath, says Dr. Andrew Weil, is the "intersection of conscious intention and primal nature and key to self-healing."[7] Controlled breathing exercises probably won't cure your cancer, I'm sorry to report, but they will almost certainly improve many cancer-related symptoms and enhance your quality of life.

Our lungs take up a majority of chest cavity real estate, which covers an area from the collarbones to the diaphragm. The mediastinum (from the Latin *mediastinus*, or "midway"), located between the lungs, contains the heart and its large blood vessels, esophagus, trachea, and lymph nodes. Mediastinum lymph node examination is an important step in the lung cancer staging process.[8]

The Lungs

Your two lungs are located on either side of the chest. The apex is the top, conical-shaped portion of the lung that fits comfortably under the collarbone. The lungs' bottom portion, or base, sits on the diaphragm. Contrary to what you may have read, the lungs aren't identical, unlike other paired organs. The right lung is typically larger than the left due to its upper, middle, and lower lobes. The smaller, left lung has just two lobes, and the "cardiac notch," a prominent, angular indentation that makes space for the heart.

Elastic fibers help the lungs expand and contract. The lungs will actually repair these fibers if they become damaged by an illness, such as chronic obstructive pulmonary disease (COPD).[9] Healthy lungs look smooth and shiny thanks to the visceral pleura, a smooth serous (watery) membrane. The parietal pleura are a membrane lining the thoracic cavity. These pulmonary pleura are slippery and slide easily over one another as the lungs expand and contract during respiration.

The bronchi are the first branch of the bronchial tree, which earned its moniker because it branches into the lungs, comprising the trachea and two primary bronchi, among other structures. The bronchi move air in and out of the lungs. As the bronchi branch, they become smaller and more numerous, just like normal tree branches. The main bronchus divides into two secondary or lobar bronchi, one for each lobe of the lung. The bronchi deliver oxygen to the lobes. From here, the airways divide into segmental bronchi, one for each lung segment.

These secondary bronchi branch several times into bronchioles, minute passageways that allow air to move through the nose or mouth to the alveoli. Atria are the final branches of the bronchial tree. They end in the alveoli, microscopic air sacs that resemble a bunch of grapes. Each lung contains approximately 300 million alveoli, which are fragile and damage easily.

Tiny blood vessels called capillaries surround the alveoli. Picture this: There are literally a billion (you heard me right) capillaries in the lungs, and extremely thin membranes separate the blood in these capillaries from the air in the alveoli. This proximity serves a purpose, allowing respiration to take place. The alveoli are the place where oxygen enters and carbon dioxide leaves the blood before being exhaled. This is why the circulatory and respiratory systems are best friends.

The lymphatics, a second important system of vessels, cross the lungs. The lungs contain a vast vessel network containing lymph, a fluid/protein mixture that's carried from the lungs and filtered before returning to the bloodstream. This vessel and lymph node system are critical to the body's immune system.[10]

Joined at the Hip: Understanding the Respiratory and Circulatory System Relationship

The Respiratory Cycle

The respiratory and circulatory systems are independent but also connected, which is why they're sometimes referred to as the "cardiorespiratory system." The respiratory system takes in oxygen and expels carbon dioxide but can't get by without the circulatory system, which it needs to distribute the oxygen. The circulatory system picks up carbon dioxide (CO_2) and waste from the tissues and delivers it to the lungs, where it's exhaled. CO_2 must be released to prevent a number of serious conditions, including hypercapnia, or excess CO_2 accumulation. Hypercapnia has many causes, including COPD, and is common in non–small cell lung cancer patients, especially those who are male, over 60 years old, and take medication.

Capillaries surrounding the alveoli pick up oxygen during the respiratory cycle. This oxygen-rich blood is transported to the heart, where arteries carry it to all body tissues. There, capillaries release oxygen and pick up carbon dioxide. Veins carry this carbon dioxide–rich blood to the heart, which pumps it to the lungs. Carbon dioxide released from the blood makes its way to the alveoli, where new oxygen is picked up before the process repeats itself. Respiratory cycle success hinges on those delicate, thin alveoli walls, which allow for the quick and easy exchange of oxygen and carbon dioxide. Lung cancer often damages the alveoli, interfering with this vital exchange of gases.

The Circulatory System

The human circulatory system is something special: an elaborate network of branched blood vessels that emanates from the heart, which moves blood throughout the body. The heart's four chambers—the right and left atrium and the right and left ventricles—work in tandem. The veins to the heart's right atrium do the dirty work, delivering CO_2-rich, O_2-poor blood from the tissues. Once in the right atrium, blood flows to the right ventricle, before leaving the heart through the pulmonary artery. Before reaching the lungs, the pulmonary artery divides into right and left branches, one for each lung. The pulmonary artery splits off several more times into arterioles, small blood vessels that branch out and keep extending and getting progressively smaller, until they reach the alveoli. These tiny, microscopic vessels are called capillaries. Only now are they capable of orchestrating the CO_2–O_2 exchange.

Blood passes through the capillaries, releasing carbon dioxide and picking up oxygen. The oxygen-rich blood gets to the left atrium via pulmonary veins. Blood passes from the left atrium into the left ventricle and is pumped out through the *aorta*, where that branching system of arteries, arterioles, and capillaries distributes it throughout the body.

Respiration: Maintaining a Delicate Balance

The human body loves equilibrium and does everything in its power to achieve and maintain balance. Respiration is referred to as a homeostatic, or stabilizing, mechanism because it simultaneously provides oxygen while removing excess carbon dioxide. But respiration is a fragile; even the smallest changes in blood oxygen or carbon dioxide levels can tip the scale, triggering an avalanche of homeostatic processes that quickly return these levels to baseline. Remember what happened the last time you went for a quick run or climbed 10 flights of stairs? All that exertion increased your breathing and heart rate. A faster heart rate speeds the rate of both oxygen delivery and carbon dioxide elimination. That quick heart rate and rapid breathing you experience after a strenuous workout are the body's expert attempt maintaining homeostasis.

You've probably heard this before, but survival is an adaptation game. Whether you realize it or not, every day your body adapts and responds to an endless array of internal and external environmental changes. This isn't a random occurrence. It's a lifesaving adaptation likely resulting from millions of years of natural selection and random mutation. Changes in the body trigger complex responses. The body's homeostatic mechanisms team up to return the internal environment to a normal state (temperature regulation, blood sugar composition, and blood pressure control are examples of homeostatic mechanisms).

Think about the kidneys for a moment. Under normal circumstances, exercise causes rapid heart and breathing rate increases (we're breathing faster in an attempt to shuttle more oxygen to our muscles). However, a limited oxygen supply causes our bodies to downshift, converting pyruvate (a molecule involved in converting sugar to energy and producing lactic acid) into something called lactate, which takes the reins and helps break down glucose, enabling energy production to continue. Lactate, or lactic acid, is a product of cell metabolism that accumulates when cells become hypoxic, meaning they lack sufficient oxygen. But this isn't a sustainable process. Muscle cells can only continue high-rate anaerobic energy production for a few minutes. High lactate levels increase muscle cell acidity, creating an unhealthy environment for the conversion of glucose to energy. In a highly acidic environment, our blood pH plummets, which triggers the kidneys to respond and assist the cardiac and respiratory systems by excreting excess acid through the urine. This is one way that different organ systems work together to maintain homeostasis.

Damaged lung tissue, like that seen in lung cancer or COPD, impairs the respiratory system's response to changes in oxygen and carbon dioxide levels, resulting in a number of serious symptoms, including shortness of breath, fatigue, dyspnea (labored breathing), and dizziness. These problems are associated with lung cancer, but they can also be symptomatic of other disorders, such as emphysema.

Pulling It All Together

The lungs are vital organs and necessary for sustaining life. They take in oxygen and expel excess carbon dioxide. Damaged lung tissue is less effective at performing the vital exchange of oxygen and carbon dioxide, leading to potentially life-altering complications.

CHAPTER 2

Cancer Fundamentals

Takeaways

- Estimates are that 8.9 million people in the United States alone are living with a cancer diagnosis.[1]
- Most cancers form tumors, but not all tumors are malignant. More tumors are benign (noncancerous), meaning they don't spread to neighboring tissues or invade other parts of the body (and probably won't kill you). Malignant tumors rage like a wildfire, invading and destroying neighboring tissues and organs.
- Few places in the body escape cancer's deadly reach. According to The National Cancer Institute, there are more than 200 cancer types, all characterized by abnormal cell growth.
- Genetic damage/change is the vehicle for transforming normal cells into cancer cells.
- All cancer cells grow abnormally and invade neighboring tissue, travel to other parts of the body, or both.
- There is no single cancer cause. Everything from chemical exposure and viruses to radiation and poor diet can cause genetic changes that contribute to the development of cancer.

Introduction

When it comes to the fight against cancer, we are most certainly living in interesting times. In fact, we're witnessing some of the greatest discoveries in the field of cancer research. Every day, it seems, we learn more and gain greater insight into the causes and development of cancer, bringing, along the way, some much-needed optimism to scientists and health care providers, not to mention the estimated millions across the globe for whom cancer is a daily part of life. I'm confident that at some point before the curtain closes on my life that we'll have in place a coordinated system to effectively prevent and treat a number of cancers, including those that kill the greatest number of people. We're getting there, but I'm not going to kid you. The road is long, and there will be unexpected twists and turns. It's going to take time. Patience isn't any easy concept to preach or teach when lives are at stake.

Patients come to my office seeking answers. Cancer is a scary illness, but most patients find learning more about their disease both empowering and reassuring. They should understand cancer and how it's treated. Knowing more about cancer keeps the all-important doctor–patient communications free and clear of static, helps patients stay on top of the latest discoveries and promising new therapies, and teaches the lost art of discernment. A discerning lung cancer patient is an empowered one.

Defining Cancer

What is cancer? A day doesn't go by that I'm not asked this question. Simply put, cancer is the uncontrolled growth of abnormal cells. We classify cancer according to abnormal cells that are growing in an abnormal way. Cancer can and does arise in nearly every part of the body, owing to the fact that, as noted earlier, there are more than 200 types of cancer, all characterized by irregular cell growth.[2]

Cancer begins in our cells. Normally, cells grow, divide, and die in a programmed, predictable way. Our cells divide only to replace old cells or to repair damage. Sometimes, however, this normal, orderly division process goes haywire and new cells form. A growth or tumor is a collection of these new, abnormal cells. Cancer cells are disease iconoclasts. They're not good at taking direction and have little regard for process and procedure. Rules mean nothing to them. They definitely follow their own game plan. Part of this, of course, is out of their control. They grow and divide with abandon, and frequently outlive their expected life span. And they form tumors. But not all tumors are cancerous. Benign tumors make better neighbors. They don't invade adjacent tissues or find their way to other body parts. Rarely do they cause serious disease, nor are they life threatening.

Malignant tumors are another story altogether. "Divide and conquer" is the malignant tumor motto. These tumors spread to neighboring tissues and organs, destroying everything in their path. They quickly spread to other body parts and regions, which is what makes them so dangerous.

Is Cancer Everywhere?

If we were to judge a disease exclusively by its ability to generate headlines, then cancer prevalence, especially in the United States, is a big deal. However, in a country of 300 million people, cancer is relatively rare. Numbers vary, but it's thought that 8.9 million people (2.6 percent of the U.S. population) will be diagnosed with cancer at some point in their lives. The American Cancer's Society's *Cancer Facts & Figures Report* states that in 2015, more than 1.6 million new cancer cases were diagnosed in the United States alone, resulting in an estimated 589,430 deaths.[3]

What Causes Cancer, Exactly?

Have you ever heard someone describe cancer cells as "abnormal"? It sounds kind of strange, but in a very real sense, they are indeed "abnormal" because they contain damaged genetic material. All human beings are born with 23 pairs of chromosomes, which contain all of the data that makes us who we are. Chromosomes, those tiny structures inside cells you may have learned about in ninth-grade biology class, consist of a substance called DNA. Every chromosome holds thousands of genes, each containing a code for a specific feature or bodily function. Your unique genetic blueprint is found in the DNA of your body's 37 trillion cells.

Genes are described in many ways, but I like to think of them as specific segments of hereditary material (DNA) that are transmitted from parent to child. Genes control our height, hair color, eye color, bone structure, and any number of other physical features. They play a role in what some people refer to as "natural" athletic ability, precocious musicality, pain tolerance, and almost certainly disease susceptibility. Genes also control cell division, repair, and death.

Every day, we're exposed to a number of things that can adversely affect our DNA. Tobacco and tobacco smoke, asbestos, radon, viruses, chemicals, and innumerable other manmade and naturally occurring toxins can cause genetic damage.[4] Our bodies are prepared for the onslaught; they're remarkably resilient, have evolved sophisticated defenses, and have built-in damage repair mechanisms. Yet, cancer may slip through the cracks, surfacing if genetic damage either overwhelms or skips by the body's normal defense and repair mechanisms. Cancer isn't an overnight process, however; it may take years of repeated attacks before a cell becomes malignant.[5]

Predictably, genes are the primary influence on cell division and cell death (apoptosis), and the process follows a precise preprogrammed time frame. Multiple mutations (damage) and a steady progression of changes at the genetic and cellular epigenetic* levels may reprogram a cell to undergo uncontrolled cell division.[6] These cells don't die. Instead, they just keep on going, forming more and more abnormal cells. This is when things turn nasty. These abnormal cells run wild, invading other tissues with reckless abandon, something their normal cell cousins would never dream of. In time, the never-say-die cancer cells overwhelm normal cells, and body functions start failing.

Cancer Cell Development: Oncogenes and Tumor Suppressor Genes

There are three classes of genes known to control cell growth and play a leading role in cancer development. Oncogenes and tumor suppressor genes are the featured performers in the development of cancer. In normal, healthy cells, proto (original)-oncogenes control cell growth and division. Oncogenes are damaged (mutated) proto-oncogenes. These damaged genes may become permanently activated or turned on, triggering uncontrolled cell production and creating a fertile environment for cancer development.[7,8]

Adenocarcinoma and squamous cell carcinoma, the most common types of non–small cell lung cancer (NSCLC), contain a number of molecular alterations, known also as "driver oncogenes." They're catalysts—troublemakers, basically—responsible both for initiating and sustaining any malignancy. About 60 percent of adenocarcinomas have driver oncogenes or oncogenes that transform normal cells into malignant cells.[9]

Normally, tumor suppressor genes (TSGs) protect against cancer by controlling cell growth.[10] TSGs are ubiquitous; we all have them. I tell my patients that tumor suppressor genes are the body's brakes, abruptly stopping cell growth and a cell's division cycle. Damage to

---

Epigenetic refers to heritable changes in gene expression that do not involve underlying changes to DNA. Such changes can happen naturally, but they are also influenced by factors such as age, lifestyle, and disease.

these genes can trigger metastases. Environmental toxins and radiation exposure can damage normal TSGs, although abnormal tumor suppressor genes can also be inherited. p53, a common TSG, regulates cell proliferation and plays a role in cell death. Damage to p53 is seen in more than 50 percent of NSCLC and more than 80 percent of small cell lung cancer (SCLC) cases.[11]

As we learn more about the changes that facilitate lung cancer cell growth, new drugs targeting these changes emerge almost daily. These drugs work differently from standard chemotherapy, sometimes working better than standard chemotherapy drugs and with fewer severe side effects. At this time, they're most often used to treat advanced lung cancers, either in conjunction with chemo or as standalone treatment.[12] I discuss targeted therapies more in Chapter 5.

What Is Cell Differentiation, and Why Should We Care About It?

As normal cells reach maturity, they "specialize" so that they can perform specific functions. Cell differentiation is another way of describing this "maturation" process. A newly differentiated lung, kidney, or liver cell looks and behaves like normal lung, kidney, and liver cell cousins. The more a cell differentiates, the more specialized it becomes and the more limited it becomes in what it can or cannot do.

Abnormal cell growth is unpredictable and inexorable; it can begin at any point during a cellular differentiation, and once the ball starts rolling, all subsequent cells will also be undifferentiated. As cancer cells grow and divide, they produce fewer and fewer differentiated cells. Less differentiated cells lose their way, to the point where they're incapable of performing tissue-specific functions.

"Differentiation" also describes the appearance of tumor cells compared with normal cells from their tissue of origin. *Well-differentiated tumors* contain cells resembling the original tissue's normal cells. *Undifferentiated tumors* cells don't resemble normal cells at all. According to cancer.gov, there's a relationship between poor cell differentiation and reduced survival among NSCLC patients with Stage I tumors.[13]

How Cancer Spreads

The ability to invade adjacent tissues and spread to remote sites is a defining cancer cell characteristic. Cancer cells are tireless road warriors. They also have a touch of attention deficit disorder and are easily bored. Once firmly ensconced in another locale, they grab a suitcase and hit the road again, traveling via the blood or lymphatic system to another part of the body where they repeat the process of growing and metastasizing all over again.

Cancers are classified according to their home tissue, not the tissues to which they metastasized. When cancer cells spread to new tissue, perhaps spurring the growth of a secondary tumor, it's still the same players, only now they're wearing the rival uniform. Lung cancer *spreads* frequently trigger brain, bone, and liver tumors. Again, these aren't new tumors. The original cancer has simply sought out a new home in a different part of the body.

Pulling It All Together

All cancer cells display uncontrolled growth and can spread to either tissues in close proximity or to areas significantly removed from the site where the cancer initially developed.[14] The trigger for cancer cell formation is genetic damage or change. Such damage or change can be fueled by exposure to environmental chemicals, toxins, and radiation and their interplay with one's inborn genetic code.

More than a million Americans have been diagnosed with cancer annually in recent years. More than 400,000 Americans with cancer have died each year. Cancer is one of the top two causes of death in this nation, and it takes the lives of some 25 percent of all Americans. We must act to alter this tragedy.

Step I
Increase Awareness

CHAPTER 3

Your Lung Cancer Primer

Takeaways

- "Lung cancer is the leading cause of cancer death and the second most common cancer among both men and women in the United States," according to the U.S. Centers for Disease Control and Prevention. More than 158,000 people in the United States and more than one million people worldwide die of lung cancer each year.
- Lung cancer can happen in any part of the lung, but up to 95 percent of lung cancer cases arise in abnormal epithelial cells in the lungs' airways. Epithelial cells cover the surface of the body and line body cavities.
- There are two major lung cancer types: small cell lung cancer (SCLC) and the far more common non–small cell (NSCLC). They have different growth patterns and require different treatments. Carcinoid tumors and malignant pleural mesothelioma are two other known cancers that may affect the lungs.
- Lung cancer type matters. Your chances for a positive outcome increase as you learn more about your disease and the available treatment options.

Introduction

For both patient and practitioner alike, there are few things more ominous than a lung cancer diagnosis. It's just awful, simple as that. Issues surface, often with an extraordinary ferocity. Supportive friends and family are an invaluable resource, but as Joseph Conrad once said, "We live as we dream—alone." The cancer journey is, in many ways, a solitary ordeal, and you may struggle to cope with the emotional effects of having lung cancer. Consider this chapter a lifeline, a vehicle to guide you down the path to receiving the best treatment. It's a comprehensive overview of all things lung cancer, including risk factors, development, growth, and spread.

How Common Is Lung Cancer?

Lung cancer accounts for more than 25 percent of all annual American cancer deaths,[1] and some 225,000 new cases are diagnosed here each year. It causes more deaths than any other particular cancer, both in this nation and worldwide. More than a million people around the globe succumb to lung cancer each year.[2]

Lung Cancer Trends

Although lung cancer is the leading killer among all forms of cancer, its significant impact is a relatively new phenomenon, thanks to the cigarette. People have used tobacco for centuries. The Mayans smoked pipes filled with tobacco and leaf resins following their evening meals. A Huron Indian myth speaks of a woman sent forth by the Great Spirit to save humanity. As she traveled the world, potatoes sprouted wherever her right hand touched the soil. Corn grew where her left hand touched the soil. Once there were sufficient amounts of corn and potatoes and the earth was rich and fertile, the woman rested. When she finally stood up, tobacco grew. Until the early 20th century, tobacco was most often chewed or smoked in a pipe or cigar. Mass cigarette production began in the late nineteenth century but didn't catch on in the United States until American GIs returned home from Europe after serving in World War I. During the war, tobacco companies donated free cigarettes to soldiers. No one anticipated the long-term impact of cigarette smoking on public health.[3]

Often I'm asked how long it takes lung cancer to develop after a person begins smoking. That's an almost impossible question to answer. Do you smoke two cigarettes a day, or two packs a day? What is your genetic makeup? What additional environmental toxins are you exposed to? Multiple factors may play a role. Surprisingly, fewer than 15 percent of lifelong smokers will get lung cancer. An even smaller percentage will contract the long list of other tobacco-related cancers, including throat or oral cancers. Part of me is hesitant to share these statistics; the fact that a majority of smokers dodge cancer doesn't diminish my desire to shepherd an effective antismoking campaign, and it should give current smokers no encouragement to continue.

Here's another way of processing the statistics: Smoking accounts for 30 percent of all cancer deaths and 87 percent of lung cancer deaths; the risk of developing lung cancer is about 23 times higher in male smokers compared with their nonsmoking counterparts; and smoking increases the risk of developing 15 different types of cancer.[4] Whenever I give a talk or presentation, I always mention that smokers live 15 years less than nonsmokers. That usually gets the audience's attention.

What does this mean? To the most obdurate smokers—those hooked on nicotine—it means a hill of beans. Doctors began to see a great increase in lung cancer during the 1930s, and by 1950, studies connected the then relatively new and widespread practice of smoking to lung cancer increases. In 1964, the very first *Surgeon General's Report on Smoking and Health* definitively declared smoking a factor in the development of lung cancer, as well as diseases including emphysema. I'm astonished, honestly, that it took the Surgeon General until 1964 to establish a link because there was existing literature detailing the cause and effect of smoking and lung cancer.[5]

Lung Cancer Doesn't Play Favorites

Is lung cancer a man's disease? It's easy to see why some people might believe that. When lung cancer incidence started increasing in the 1930s, most cases were observed in men. Starting with the returning WWI GIs, most smokers were men. The tide started turning in the 1960s, when cigarette ad campaigns began targeting women. Today, smoking rates are nearly equal for men and women.[6] The result of this unfortunate trend has been a steady increase in the incidence of lung cancer among women. Some countries have even seen lung cancer become the number one killer of women, killing more women than breast cancer.[7] The lung cancer deaths we're seeing among women are tied to 1970s smoking trends. Lung cancer takes time to develop.

Why Is Cancer Rising among Nonsmoking Women?

"How could I possibly have this?"

It's a comment I've heard more than a few times in my office. And the comment doesn't come from the mouth of a hardened, two-pack-a-day smoker, but from a stunned nonsmoking female patient. In fact, 20 percent of women who never touch a cigarette will develop lung cancer.[8] While lung cancer rates have fallen 21 percent among men—owing to early diagnosis and targeted and aggressive antismoking campaigns—rates among women jumped 116 percent between 1975 and 2012. Adding to the heartbreak, for many of these women the disease is well advanced at the time of diagnosis, limiting treatment options for cure. Early symptoms are often mistaken for the common cold. So please don't ignore that lingering cough.

Small cell lung cancer (SCLC) and non–small cell lung cancer (NSCLC) are the two major lung cancer types. Distinct subtypes, characterized by damaged genes and abnormal proteins, are other types of lung cancer. For example, young nonsmokers with lung cancer commonly have mutations in a gene called EGFR (epidermal growth factor receptor).

And there's almost certainly a hereditary basis to the disease's development, as there is with a majority of cancers.[9] Most recent science shows that in lung cancers developed before a person is 69 years old, just over 1.5 percent have a genetic component that may be shared by close relatives.

The risk of developing lung cancer doubles if a person has a parent, sibling, or child with lung cancer. This risk associated with having a first-degree relative with the disease is greater for women and nonsmokers. Having a more distant relative, such as an aunt or niece with lung cancer, increases your risk of developing the disease by about 30 percent. This genetic susceptibility, combined with other factors, including hormonal changes or exposure to cancer-causing substances such as secondhand smoke, radon, uranium, arsenic, nickel, and asbestos, may trigger the onset. Recent studies suggest that women are more susceptible to smoking's cancer-triggering effects.

While lung cancer rates have been on the rise in nonsmoking women, a Stanford University study found that, on average, female lung cancer patients with advanced stage disease survive two months longer than their male counterparts.[10] Two months might not sound like much when you're forty years old and staring at a possible life sentence, but it's significant. The same genetic differences that make women more vulnerable to cancer in the first place may be the very small factor that extends their survival rate. A woman's cells may be less efficient at repairing DNA damage, and so they more easily contract cancer. On the other hand, women's bodies appear to have an easier time ridding themselves of cancer cells. What's the answer? Who knows, but stay tuned.

Lung Cancer Risk Factors

There are a number of chemicals and environmental factors that make our internal environment a potent lung cancer breeding ground.

Smoking

In case you haven't figured it out, I detest cigarette smoking. There is no greater risk factor for lung cancer than smoking. Current and former smokers fill my waiting room and account for more than 85 percent of all lung cancer cases, according to cancer.gov.[11] Nicotine is insidious, its effects, cumulative. In other words, it's the total lifetime exposure to cigarette smoke, expressed in "pack-years" (packs per year over a number of years), that weighs most heavily when determining a person's risk of developing lung cancer. Tobacco is not the only carcinogen containing smoke. Marijuana is also filled with numerous carcinogens. Without engaging in a debate over the merits of legalization or marijuana's medicinal value, it's a fact that marijuana smoke increases a person's risk of lung cancer. Don't let anyone tell you otherwise.

Hands down, quitting is the most effective way to lower lung cancer risk. Be warned, however, that the risk doesn't drop as soon as that last pack of cigarettes finds its way to the garbage can. Lung cancer can fester for decades before symptoms surface. Still, people who quit smoking are 50 percent less likely to develop the disease than those who continue smoking. Therefore, when a patient asks "If I already have lung cancer, what's the point of quitting?" my best advice never changes: "Don't start."

"If I already have lung cancer, Dr. Presser, what's the point of quitting?"

Nihilism is another unintended, but not unexpected, consequence I see in smokers following a lung cancer diagnosis. This is nothing more than illogical thinking. If you have lung cancer, quit smoking—immediately. Ex-smokers experience fewer post-surgical complications and respond better to treatment. Ex-smokers who've been successfully treated for SCLC are less likely to develop additional lung tumors. Quitting smoking slows the progress of other lung disorders such as emphysema, bladder cancer, and other tobacco-related diseases, like mouth and stomach cancer.[12]

Smoking isn't just a bad habit. It's a physical and psychological addiction to nicotine, which meets all the established addictive drug criteria. Some studies indicate that cocaine is less addictive than nicotine and that its addictive power is equal to that of heroin, a concept reflected in popular culture with the term "nicotine junkie." A report issued by the Tobacco Advisory Group of Britain's Royal College of Physicians concluded, "Most smokers do not smoke out of choice, but because they are addicted to nicotine."[13]

There are available resources to help you quit. Nicotine patches, chewing gums, inhalers, and other nicotine replacement options are all viable therapies that can double the rates of successful smoking cessation in the first 6 to 12 months.[14] Counseling and support groups can help as well. Please see Chapter 8 for tips on quitting smoking.

Secondhand Smoke

The health risks of tobacco smoke are not limited to smokers. People in the same environment—the same house, office, car, and even outside spaces—are also exposed to the smoke's carcinogens and thus also face an increased risk of lung cancer. There are more than 400 chemicals in secondhand smoke, 50 of which are known carcinogens. The federal Environmental Protection Agency (EPA) estimates that 3,000 people in the United States die of lung cancer each year because of exposure to secondhand smoke. Children are particularly vulnerable. They're more prone to sudden infant death syndrome (SIDS), ear infections, cough, colds, and tooth decay.[15]

Environmental Carcinogens

Do environmental factors really affect cancer risk? If we're to believe the American Cancer Society (ACS), then they most certainly do.

According to the ACS, most cancer cases don't stem from inherited genes but from damage arising from environmental concerns such as poor nutrition, smoking, overweight, obesity, and physical inactivity. In fact, environmental causes are suspected in 75 to 80 percent of cancer cases and deaths in the United States (hereditary factors account for the remainder). The ACS also notes a "significant burden" from a range of environmental exposures that include 107 agents known to being central to human cancer development, including, but not limited to tobacco, asbestos, and radiation. These environmental carcinogens are substances that can cause genetic damage or produce epigenetic changes that contribute to cancer development. Because I'm a bit out of my element here, I recruited my friend and colleague, Dr. Stewart Lonky, a Los Angeles–based pulmonologist and nationally recognized expert on environmental toxins, to compile a list of the most lethal lung carcinogens.

Asbestos   Asbestos is a natural, fibrous mineral and, for many years, a manufacturing and construction industry staple made popular, in part, by its heat resistance. "Asbestos exposure increases the risk for lung cancer and malignant pleural mesothelioma, a rare form of cancer involving the covering of the lungs. Mesothelioma always is asbestos related," says Dr. Lonky. "Everyone has some low-level exposure to asbestos and depending on the cumulative dose, when combined with other variables, asbestos is potentially a cancer risk factor for everyone, not just smokers. Also, asbestos is a co-carcinogen; that is, if you combine it with smoking you have a 100-times increased risk," he adds. Because lung cancer can appear decades after exposure, it's imperative for those exposed to first- or secondhand smoke to be checked every five years. Dr. Lonky warns that people living with workers who are exposed to asbestos are at risk as well.

Benzene   Benzene made headlines recently after a methane gas well leak in the upscale Los Angeles suburb of Porter Ranch. Following the leak, higher than normal benzene levels were detected in air samples. Benzene is a colorless, sweet-smelling petroleum and coal component that's used to make plastics, lubricants, dyes, adhesives, and pesticides. It's also a key ingredient in cigarettes and, not surprisingly, is the 17th most produced chemical in the United States, according to the Center for Public Integrity website. "Benzene is a known human carcinogen and it's been linked to a number of

cancers," says Dr. Lonky. The liver releases metabolites, the byprod-
ucts of metabolized benzene, after benzene has entered the body via
inhaled vapors. Inhaled benzene irritates the linings of the airways.
"High-level exposure can severely damage the lungs, causing fluid
accumulation and bleeding, which is often fatal," says Dr. Lonky.

Radon   Radon is an invisible, cancer-causing radioactive gas. Indeed,
radon exposure may be the root cause of 15,000 to 22,000 lung cancer deaths in the United States annually, according to EPA estimates.[16]
Radon isn't ubiquitous, however. Concentrations vary considerably.
"Miners and other underground workers, as an example, may
be exposed to high levels of radon in uranium-rich areas," says
Dr. Lonky. High ground levels of radon can trigger high levels of in-
door exposure, which explains the popularity of home testing kits.
Dealing with bureaucracies is never fun, but if you're concerned
about radon levels in your home, you may also want to contact your
local public health department.

Arsenic   In literature and movies, arsenic ranks up there with hem-
lock and cyanide as an effective way to bump someone off. Arsenic is
a naturally occurring element found in the earth's crust. It's found in
both inorganic and organic forms, but only the inorganic form is a
known carcinogen. Not surprisingly, inorganic arsenic found its way
into insecticide production and a number of other lethal products,
including weed killers, rat poison, fungicides, and wood preserva-
tives. Arsenic also turns up in some paints and leather industry pre-
servatives. "It's everywhere, really," Dr. Lonky observes, and, as such,
"there's no way to avoid it altogether," he adds. Mining, copper
smelting, and pesticide manufacturing or application can—and often
do—put people at great risk of inorganic arsenic exposure.[17] We're
also exposed to arsenic when we use rice-based products.

Bisphenol A   Bisphenol A (BPA), a polycarbonate plastic building
block, is one of the most widely manufactured chemicals in the world.
Accordingly, it's found in toys, cell phones, receipts printed on thermal
paper, most food and beverage container linings, and dozens of other
consumer products. BPA is a known "endocrine disruptor," meaning it
interferes with the body's endocrine system, affecting growth, behavior, reproduction, and development. Although a study found that low
doses of BPA do not cause any ill health effects, it was also found in
laboratory studies to "stimulate lung cancer cell migration."

Chromium Odorless and colorless, this naturally occurring element is ubiquitous, turning up in rocks, animals, plants, and soil. It exists in several forms, but one in particular, chromium VI, or hexavalent chromium, is carcinogenic. "Exposure to hexavalent chromium increases risk for developing lung cancer, no doubt about it," points out Dr. Lonky. Chrome plating, stainless steel welding, and chromium-nickel foundry work are occupations that increase risk of chromium (VI) exposure.[18] It's especially heavy in water, soil, and foods.

Dioxins "Dioxin" refers to a group of chemically related compounds that are known endocrine disrupters and persistent organic pollutants (POP). They settle in animal fatty tissue and degrade slowly. Most human dioxin exposure comes through food such as shellfish, dairy, and meat. Dioxins accumulate in fat cells and degrade very slowly in the environment. "Since they're in both the endocrine disruptor and POP categories, they're almost certainly at the root of reproductive and developmental problems, immune system suppression, increased heart disease and diabetes rates, and many different cancer types," Dr. Lonky says. Although a number of studies show an increased lung cancer risk from dioxin exposure, the specific risk is no greater than other cancers linked to occupational dioxin exposure.

Nickel This compound of silvery-white metal used to make stainless steel and other metal alloys has been shown to increase the risk for lung and nasal sinus cancers. Metalworking, nickel mining and smelting, sandblasting, stainless steel manufacturing, paint and varnish manufacturing, and welding are just a partial list of the occupations that can potentially expose a person to unsafe amounts of nickel.[19] "Nickel exposure in the general population, which comes from jewelry and stainless steel, isn't usually high enough to be of concern for most people. However, in workplaces where nickel compounds are produced and used, the risk is much greater," says Dr. Lonky.

Polycyclic Aromatic Hydrocarbons "Just awful," says Dr. Lonky about this lethal group of chemicals that forms during the incomplete burning of coal, oil, gas, garbage, or other organic substances, such as tobacco or charbroiled meat. Diesel fuel exhaust is a prevalent source of polycyclic aromatic hydrocarbons (PAHs), for example. "PAHs are potent carcinogens, and they're found everywhere, increasing our susceptibility to a host of breathing and lung-related illnesses, including lung cancer," warns Dr. Lonky. Tobacco smoke, wood smoke, vehicle exhaust, asphalt roads, and agricultural burn smoke all contain high levels of PAHs, as do tar, crude oil, creosote, and roofing tar. Some PAHs are used to make medicines, dyes, plastics, and pesticides. Other sources include coal gasification, petroleum refineries, asphalt and pavement work, roofing, and aluminum production.[20,21] PAHs attach themselves to micro particles, and they get inhaled or consumed by the animals we consume. Animal and plant PAH concentrations are much higher and create free-radical damage and turn off our cancer-protective mechanisms.

Other Environmental Lung Carcinogens   There are other, less known but equally lethal lung carcinogens. These include ether, chloromethyl methyl ether, ionizing radiation (X-rays), gamma radiation, mustard gas, soot, tars, mineral oils, and vinyl chloride. Suspected lung carcinogens include acrylonitrile, cadmium, beryllium, lead, and ferric oxide dust, among others.

Genetic Factors

Have you ever seen people walking around the streets, particularly in large, overpopulated cities, with masks covering their noses and mouths? These don't do much good, sorry to say. We've done a pretty good job of poisoning our air, not to mention the soil and water. At this point, we're all subjected to a fair number of lung carcinogens. Exposure totals are one factor governing lung cancer development, but by no means are they the only factor. The normal to malignant cancer cell transformation is a variable, multistep process.[22] Thus, it's not only what we're exposed to, but also how our bodies process the onslaught that determines whether lung cancer takes hold of our lives.

Genes control how our bodies deal with carcinogens and determine our susceptibility to carcinogen-related disease and how effectively we repair the damage. Our genes also control our immune system's ability to detect and destroy cancer cells. There are some folks who seem to be at increased risk of developing lung cancer, irrespective of their lifestyle habits, and others who are seemingly resistant to the effects of carcinogens. I happen to have treated a number of lifelong smokers for issues other than lung cancer, as well as a number of nonsmokers who died from the disease. Lung cancer cells contain a significant number of genetic changes. It's not uncommon to find 10 to 20 genetic mutations, indicating a genetic instability in lung cancer cells.[23]

Age

Because 80 percent of cancer cases occur in people over age 60,[24] age certainly contributes to a person's lung cancer risk. Two-thirds of lung cancer patients are age 65 or older at the time of diagnosis; the average age of newly diagnosed patients is 70. Genetic damage is a cumulative event; it may take multiple defects before a cell becomes cancerous. And as we age, our immune system, like others among our biological systems, weakens, so cancer cells become more likely to slip in and grow.[25]

Lung Cancer Growth

Lung cancer is a slow grower, for the most part. A lung tumor that reaches one centimeter in diameter (approximately three-eighths of an inch) is already an older cancer and may have been present for up to 15 years. This isn't to say that all lung cancers grow slowly; there is variability in tumor growth. An interesting report from the International Early Lung Cancer Action Program (ELCAP) found that the growth rates for lung cancer detected following repeated rounds of yearly computed tomography (CT) screening were not "significantly different from growth rates reported for cancers diagnosed in clinical practice in the absence of screening." In a press release, the ELCAP also said the frequencies of small-cell carcinoma and adenocarcinoma among all lung cancers were approximately 20 percent and 50 percent, respectively, without screening. After repeated rounds of CT screening, these numbers were nearly identical at 19 percent and 50 percent.[26] Although the majority of lung cancers grow slowly, they all possess the ability to metastasize or spread to other body parts, a process known as early micrometastasis.[27] Heavy blood flow through the highly vascularized lungs certainly facilitates and even speeds up the metastatic process. Though some tumors grow slowly, the larger the growth, the greater the chance it's invaded neighboring tissue or spread.

How Lung Cancer Spreads

Lung cancer cells aren't as tough as you may have read or as many of us have been led to believe. Most that enter the bloodstream die quickly, killed off by our body's natural defense mechanisms. However, those lung cancer cells from the original tumor site that enter the blood steam and somehow survive the treacherous journey will take up residence at another site away from the lungs, resulting in new tumor growth.

The lungs are fertile ground for cancer. Vascularization provides a vast network of cancer-friendly routes for tumor cells to travel to other body parts. The lungs' lymphatic vessels, part of the body's immune system, may trap some cancer cells, which then multiply, causing swelling (i.e., lymph node enlargement). This is why a thorough workup will include an examination of the lymph nodes in a patient's chest. Such examination can determine whether cancer cells have moved beyond the main tumor and to other parts of the body, causing further tumors in those regions. This is where staging becomes so critical. Staging, or the extent of disease spread, is perhaps the single biggest variable in helping determine a patient's treatment options.

Three factors determine cancer stage:

- How large is the original or primary tumor, and what are its characteristics?
- Has the cancer spread to adjacent lymph nodes? (Regional lymph node involvement may indicate spread to distant areas of the body.) If it has spread, where, and how many nodes are involved?
- Are there any distant metastases? In other words, has the primary tumor spread to other parts of the body, leading to secondary tumor development?

Types of Lung Cancer

How do we determine lung cancer type? Historically, oncologists have classified lung cancer based on how it looks under a microscope. Today, however, there are supplemental tests that help pathologists diagnosis lung cancer subtypes, explaining the flux in lung cancer classification (the World Health Organization provides the classification scheme).[28]

SCLC and NSCLC are the two primary lung cancers. NSCLC accounts for 85 percent of all lung cancers; the remaining 15 percent are SCLC.[29] These are different diseases; their growth and spread patterns vary, and so do treatment options.

Non–Small Cell Lung Cancer

NSCLC accounts for 85 percent of all lung cancer cases. Adenocarcinoma, squamous cell carcinoma, and large cell carcinoma are the three primary types of NSCLC. They're named for the sorts of cells found in the tumor and how they behave. There are variants or subtypes of the primary cancers as well, the names of which describe certain microscopic growth patterns. The following section briefly describes the defining features of NSCLC.

Adenocarcinoma   Although overall lung cancer rates have dropped in the past 20 years, adenocarcinoma rates have gone up, especially in women.[30] Lifestyle factors including smoking, dietary pattern and habits, and environmental and occupational exposures all are thought to play a role.

Adenocarcinoma is the most common primary cancer type, accounting for an estimated 40 percent of all lung cancers in the United States and approximately 55 percent of NSCLCs. Adenocarcinoma is the most common lung cancer in nonsmokers, and the most common lung cancer type diagnosed in people under age 50. In situ pulmonary adenocarcinoma (AIS), previously called bronchioloalveolar adenocarcinoma, is an adenocarcinoma subtype that has a slow growth pattern and is less likely to metastasize than other forms of NSCLC, offering the possibility of a more favorable outcome.[31]

Squamous Cell Carcinoma   The numbers are down, but that hasn't stopped squamous cell carcinoma (SCC) from retaining the dubious distinction as the most common lung cancer type among current and former smokers. SCC makes up 25 percent of all lung cancers. Unlike adenocarcinoma, SCC is diagnosed more in men and in folks over age 65, who already make up a fair percentage of the lung cancer demographic. SCC tumors are frequently found in the central area of the lung and, like bronchioloalveolar adenocarcinoma, grow slowly, metastasizing later than other forms of NSCLC.[32] Although they don't generally spread to distant sites, these tumors are just as pesky and habitually invade neighboring structures.

Large Cell Carcinoma   Large cell carcinoma (LCC) has been assigned the moniker of "baby tumor" because it may just be an immature adenocarcinoma or squamous cell carcinoma. LCC turns up in 10 to 15 percent of U.S. lung cancer cases and can surface anywhere in the lung. LCC is bad news, as it's an active and aggressive form of NSCLC.[33,34]

Small Cell Lung Cancer

As the name implies, SCLC is a *small* cancer, which explains why it's sometimes referred to as "oat cell carcinoma." SCLC is a highly malignant cancer that most commonly arises in the lung. Compared with NSCLC, SCLC has a shorter doubling time, higher growth rate, and spreads earlier to distant sites.

Here are a few SCLC facts and characteristics

- Tobacco smoking is the biggest risk factor for SCLC: 98 to 99 percent of patients with SCLC have a long history of tobacco use.[35] Radon gas exposure is also a risk factor for SCLC.
- SCLC metastasizes quickly, spreading to mediastinal lymph nodes, liver, bones, adrenal glands, and brain.
- Although 60 to 90 percent of SCLC patients initially respond well to chemotherapy and radiation, there's a very high relapse rate with this type of cancer. In 60 to 70 percent of SCLC patients, the disease has spread beyond the primary tumor site at the time of diagnosis.[36]
- SCLC often surfaces in the bronchi (airways), near the center of the chest.
- At the time of diagnosis, SCLC has typically spread to distant sites.

Other Lung Cancers

Carcinoid Tumors

This is a rare, slow-growing tumor that accounts for a small percentage (1–5 percent) of all lung cancers. They're seen most often in people under 40 but are equally common in men and women. They start frequently in the digestive tract or lungs, although there's no established relationship between smoking and carcinoid tumors. Because carcinoid tumors originate in neuroendocrine cells, which are specialized hormone-producing nerve cells, they secrete lots of hormones, leading to symptoms such as diarrhea and flushing. Carcinoid tumors don't often spread beyond local lymph nodes, however. Atypical carcinoid tumors are an aggressive carcinoid tumor variant that are more likely to spread and reoccur than garden-variety carcinoid tumors.[37]

Malignant Pleural Mesothelioma

Malignant pleural mesothelioma (MPM) is a cancer of the lining of the lungs (pleura) but can also originate in the abdomen or the sac around the heart or testes. MPM is seen after prolonged exposure to asbestos

(asbestos is the leading cause of MPM). Mesothelioma develops in the pleura, the tissue covering the lungs and internal chest wall. (75 percent of malignant mesotheliomas occur in the pleura of the lungs, a common metastatic cancer site). There are an estimated 2,000 to 3,000 new malignant mesothelioma cases in the United States each year.[38] Many factors determine treatment options. Chemotherapy, surgery, radiation therapy, or a combination may be offered, depending on the extent of the disease, a person's age, and other underlying medical issues. Many doctors do not ask about asbestos exposure, and diagnosis is often delayed. For example, if you've had fluid drained from your chest more than once, your doctor may recommend VATS to obtain tissue for a definitive diagnosis.

Pulling It All Together

By far, smoking is the single greatest risk factor for lung cancer, accounting for 80 percent of deaths in men and 90 percent in women. Men who smoke are 23 times more likely to develop lung cancer. Women are 13 times more likely, compared with those who've never smoked. Thus, if you smoke, the best advice is to take steps to quit—immediately.

Still, the rise in lung cancer among nonsmokers—or more accurately, never-smokers—is disconcerting. For example, according to a study presented at the 16th World Conference on Lung Cancer in 2015, the incidence of never-smokers diagnosed with NSCLC jumped from 13 to 28 percent during a six-year period. Of greatest concern, a number of these patients presented with advanced-stage disease.

Although antismoking strategies implemented in the late 1970s and early 1980s have led to a decrease in the number of smoking-related lung cancer cases, the rise in lung cancer rates among non-smokers and never-smokers is concerning. So what is causing never-smokers to develop lung cancer?

Step II

Get a Proper Diagnosis

CHAPTER 4

Diagnosing and Staging Lung Cancer

Takeaways

- "Staging" lung cancer means determining whether the cancer is confined to the lungs or has spread to other sites.
- Lung cancer isn't an overnight process. Tumors often grow for a long time before they're detected. When common symptoms such as coughing and fatigue occur, people dismiss them, understandably thinking they stem from other causes, which makes early lung cancer go undiagnosed. Lung cancer may be the most common cancer worldwide, but it's still far less widespread than a cold, flu, or bronchitis. Most people with lung cancer are not diagnosed until, at best, Stage III, and this fact buttresses the argument for low-dose computed tomography (CT) screening for those at greatest risk.
- Staging is basically broken down into three categories. The anatomic stage, starting with the letter "T," describes the size of the primary or original tumor. There are two prognostic groups, "N," which indicates any lymph node involvement, and "M," or "metastasis," which indicates whether the cancer has spread. Staging begins with an "occult carcinoma," which is a primary tumor that cannot be assessed, or a tumor proven by the presence of malignant cells but not seen with imaging or a bronchoscopy. The next stages are Stage IA, Stage IB, Stage IIA, Stage IIB, Stage IIIA, Stage IIIB, and Stage IV. Stage IV indicates that cancer has spread throughout the body.

Introduction

Health is a tricky thing. We don't give it much thought unless there's an obvious symptom, indicating that something is wrong. Who thinks about their eyesight until they can't see or their feet until they can't walk? Sadly, some people think they're in great shape only to find out that they have a serious medical condition or disease.

Our lungs fall into this category. They're vital organs, providing our bodies with life-sustaining oxygen while eliminating carbon dioxide. Healthy lungs are resilient; they have to be. They're tasked with meeting the human body's almost insatiable need for oxygen even under the most trying circumstances. Think about the lung capacity needed to complete a triathlon or sing an opera. Unless you're gasping for breath after climbing a short flight of stairs, however, you're not going to give your lungs much thought.

You know the expression, "What doesn't kill you makes you stronger"? When it comes to the lungs, what makes you stronger sometimes kills you. It is, in fact, the lungs' resiliency that allows tumors to flourish even for years without any adverse effect on lung function. Somehow they carry on, even under the most trying circumstances. Because the lungs also have fewer nerves than other organs, it's easy to see how someone can have lung cancer, but remain asymptomatic for many years. This is why a majority of patients don't receive a diagnosis until the disease has moved beyond the primary or original tumor site. With no pain felt for potentially years as the tumor grows, the cancer can spread silently, making it difficult if not impossible to cure. Lung cancer patients aren't asymptomatic, but the symptoms occur later in the disease process, or they're dismissed as stemming from another, far less serious illness. In the world of medicine, lung cancer is truly a "silent killer."

Concern over lung cancer's long silent growth pattern has generated some buzz around the subject of screening. I routinely field questions about the subject. This chapter looks at the value and necessity of lung cancer screening, lung cancer diagnosis, and staging—the processes that determine cancer spread and extent.

I begin with a true story about the value of early detection. As you'll learn from my patient Jack's lung cancer journey, screening is perhaps the single most important thing you can do to catch the disease early, particularly if you're at risk. Estimates are that 85 percent of lung cancer patients receive a positive diagnosis only after symptoms develop, meaning that a majority of patients have advanced-stage disease. A key component of the prevention model is the widespread availability of a concerted lung cancer–screening program. It's my deepest conviction that if such a program were instituted, we'd shatter the late-stage diagnosis pattern.

Jack's Story

Around the courts of his Los Angeles tennis club, Jack was something of a legend—"85 going on 40" is how his regular doubles partners described him. An ex-Marine, Jack approached his thrice-weekly tennis games with the same zeal he displayed while defending his country during the Korean War. So Jack kept going, even at an age when most people give up sports for a more sedentary life. Even the niggling, avoidable injuries that challenge most tennis players didn't deter Jack or diminish his enthusiasm. So when he fell while chasing down a shot, he didn't give it much thought. It's not like this hadn't happened before. "An occupational hazard," Jack would joke with his tennis buddies. As a soldier and two-sport athlete in college, Jack was used to falling, but save for a bruised body part or ego, it was generally a benign event. Certainly, it was nothing that could cause a life-threatening injury. But on one especially warm June morning, it nearly did. Within hours of falling, Jack's entire left side was black and blue; every breath caused excruciating pain because Jack's aging bones had been fractured, a painful and serious injury in an older adult.

Jack's wife, a former intensive care nurse and chronic worrier, immediately suspected broken ribs and demanded that he make an appointment with his primary care physician. Of course, Jack didn't want to. Marines are nothing if not self-sufficient and used to "toughing it out," as he liked to tell his grandkids. Another reason for Jack's reluctance had to do with his long-abandoned smoking habit, which he picked up following his stint in the service. The residual effect of a 25-year, pack-a-day habit doesn't just disappear overnight.

After two days of nonstop wifely nudging, which Jack confided was worse than the pain in his chest, he reluctantly scheduled an appointment with his internist. The following day, Jack was in his doctor's office, his worrying wife close by his side. After briefly examining his patient, Jack's doctor ordered a chest X-ray, standard procedure for anyone age 85 with a long history of smoking and extensive bruising. The X-ray revealed a single spot in his right lung. A solitary round spot on a chest X-ray, often referred to as a lung nodule, could be an early sign of cancer, although nodules are common and just as often benign. Still, given Jack's age and medical history, his doctor ordered a computed tomography (CT) scan.

In medicine, where there's smoke, there's usually fire, and the CT revealed a mass in the right lower lobe of Jack's lung. As a rule, the smaller the nodule, the less likely it may be cancerous. A nodule that measures less than .05 cm, or about one-fifth of an inch, for example, is extremely likely to be benign. On the other hand, nodules measuring more than 2 cm, which is about three-quarters of an inch, have a greater than 50 percent likelihood of being cancerous. Jack's lung mass measured 4 cm. A needle biopsy was performed to obtain a sample of this suspicious-looking lung nodule. This was the least invasive way to sample the mass in Jack's lung—no small consideration given his age.

The test results confirmed Jack's worst fear: lung cancer, specifically adenocarcinoma, the most common form. Fortunately for Jack, a subsequent positron emission tomography (PET) scan showed that the tumor hadn't spread, making surgery the best option. But Jack's first surgical consult didn't go well at all. "Jack, I have to be honest. I think you're too old to undergo an operation to remove the tumor," said the doctor. Jack's heart sank. His wife started sobbing uncontrollably. Unbeknownst to Jack and his wife, his doctor, a traditional thoracic surgeon, didn't perform minimally invasive surgery. He only used conventional methods, which require larger incisions, a longer hospital stay and recovery, and prolonged pain.

Jack was confused. He was an ex-Marine corporal who exercised regularly and followed a healthy diet; he didn't feel like he was 85. He was used to getting things done. "Never take no for an answer," he'd tell his troops. Now, he was in another fight for his life. He had cancer and wanted it out—no questions asked. "Too old" was the last thing he wanted to hear.

Jack sought a second opinion with me. From the moment of our initial consultation, I knew Jack was a fighter. After years of heavy combat in the Korean War, he felt as though cancer was a walk in the park. Jack came to my office searching for answers and for hope because he'd heard that I do minimally invasive thoracic surgery. I explained that lung cancer is always treatable, but given the diagnosis of Stage I cancer, our goal was cure. I promised Jack that before he left my office, we'd have a plan in place.

I led Jack out of the exam room back to my office so we could review the CT scan of his chest. With lung spots, a picture is truly worth a thousand words. Rather than scaring Jack and his wife, the picture on the screen helped them understand the nature of his condition.

Surgery is most commonly done as treatment for early-stage lung cancer. Once it's spread, early stage non–small cell lung cancer is better treated with chemotherapy and/or radiation initially. From Jack's CT scan, it didn't appear to me that his cancer had spread to his lymph nodes, which a subsequent PET scan confirmed. When used in conjunction, a PET scan gives a clearer picture about how lung cancer should be treated. Unlike a CT scan, which looks at the body anatomically, PET scans pick up biological changes. Because cells use sugar for food, a small amount of radioactive sugar is injected into the bloodstream before the scan. Rapidly growing cancer cells devour the sugar and can be seen on imaging. With lung cancer, we need to know how far the cancer has advanced to determine the best course of treatment. Studies suggest that using the results of a PET scan along with a CT scan improves staging accuracy. If Jack's lung cancer had spread to distant lymph nodes, surgery would not have been the first treatment option.

Jack fell into the category of "resection for cure," and because I could perform this procedure with minimally invasive surgical techniques, his age and state of health weren't mitigating factors. I would remove a four-centimeter mass from Jack's right lung. Because we already knew it was a cancer mass, I would also resect his entire right lower lobe and the appropriate lymph nodes, which would help stage his cancer. Jack's wife started to cry. She gently gripped the hand of the man she'd been married to for almost 60 years. I could see that Jack's mood had changed as well. *No one likes to see me.* But on this warm June morning, I took comfort in helping make an unpleasant process manageable.

The next time I saw Jack and his wife was on the morning of his operation. Changing into a hospital gown is one of the most traumatic parts of preparing for surgery. We exchanged pleasantries, and I answered many of the same questions again. Jack apologized. I told him there are no dumb questions. "I do this every day, and you're doing this once." That always brings a smile to patients' faces. As the surgical nurse wheeled Jack into the operating room, I reassured his wife that she would see her husband cancer free. She knew I meant it.

As lung cancer surgery goes, Jack's procedure was uneventful. The minimally invasive surgery allowed him to return home just three days later. When I saw Jack one week later in my office for a follow-up visit, he informed me that he'd gone bowling with a group of friends and was back to his normal self, pain free. I smiled. I explained to Jack that the lymph nodes I removed were cancer free. "That's great. Now what?" he asked. "You're cancer free. Go enjoy your life. Leave the worrying to your wife and me." At his three-month follow-up, Jack told me that he'd never felt better, still plays tennis and has a renewed enthusiasm for chasing after his six grandchildren. This life-altering experience has helped me realize that things I once thought were important really aren't. Each day is a blessing.

I was relieved for Jack and his family, but many stories don't turn out as well. Patients die, particularly when the disease has advanced past the lungs and local lymph nodes. But I did say that every condition is treatable. What's the difference? I tell every one of my patients that our work together is all about living. They don't have cancer. They are people living *with* cancer. I encourage my patients to continue with the business of their lives, so long as they're feeling up to it, grave diagnosis notwithstanding. I try to care for their emotional needs and give them tools to help endure the journey. My patients are my second family. I get to know them on a personal level. Why shouldn't I? They're putting their lives in my hands. The close personal relationship is our bond. I have their back.

"Hope is everything," I tell my patients. Of course, I'd like to think that having a good doctor helps, but without hope, there's nothing. As one patient told me years ago during my residency, "Whatever you do, don't take away my hope because without hope, I have nothing." You can apply that statement to so many scenarios. With lung cancer, it's all about hope and living. It's important to know, however, that work isn't about false hope. It's about hope. It's about the idea that "we're a team. And we're going to get through this together."

Jack's story is a classic cautionary tale about the value of early detection and screening. His postfall chest X-ray, which led to a CT scan, literally saved his life. This is the value of screening, particularly for an ex-smoker like Jack. Although in this case I wouldn't have performed a needle biopsy, there is no one-size-fits-all model for diagnosing and treating lung cancer. Clinical scenarios vary, but what's constant is that patients need answers. They need to know what to do if a lung mass is found. The bottom line is diagnosis is absolutely paramount in forming a proper treatment plan, and every patient needs to know his or her options.

Lung Cancer Screening and Early Detection

Any dialogue about lung cancer diagnosis must begin with a discussion of screening. Healthy or sick, it doesn't matter. Screening is useful for detecting lung cancer in people at risk and even in seemingly healthy people with no symptoms at all who may have unrecognized cancer or precancerous changes in the lung. Screening identifies the disease early, allowing doctors to proactively treat lung cancer, improve patient prognosis, and increase the chances of long-term survival. As importantly, screening allows those with precancerous changes to take steps so the disease never materializes and offers peace of mind to those at risk—or to anyone interested in taking charge of his or her health.

It struck me as odd that until 2013, there was no formal lung cancer screening program. What took so long?

Despite mounting evidence to the contrary, people still believe that lung cancer only happens to smokers and is thus a behaviorally based disease. If those damn smokers hadn't lit up in the first place, they never would have gotten lung cancer.

The fact that lung cancer grows slowly and can be asymptomatic for decades hasn't helped the screening cause. Remember what I said earlier? When it comes to our health, we fix the wagon after the wheels have fallen off.

A recent study suggesting that the lung cancer diagnosis rate is the same, with or without screening, has further muddied the waters, and there are even a handful of physicians who question the value of screening. Some have raised issue with the potential harms from screening, including repeated or prolonged radiation exposure, incidental findings, misdiagnosis, and false positives. Evidence from the 2011 National Lung Screening Trial (NLST) found that almost 25 percent of patients screened by CT had positive results, but more than 95 percent of those did not ultimately receive a cancer diagnosis. Others worry that scans also find cancers that don't really matter. Some cancers grow slowly, so much so that they never really pose a threat. Twenty-five percent of the NLST participants had multiple tests showing abnormal growths in the lungs that turned out be benign. False-positive tests can lead to costly and even risky procedures like biopsies.[1]

My argument to the critics is "so what?" In my estimation, the value of screening far outweighs the risks. In an important opinion piece in *The New York Times,* Andrea McKee, chairwoman of the department of radiation oncology at Lahey Hospital and Medical Center, and Andrew Salner, radiation oncology chief at Hartford Hospital, observed, "There is, increasingly, a consensus that CT screening for lung cancer can save thousands of lives each year."[2] The same NLST also found that low-dose CT scanning is effective for detecting early-stage lung cancer and potentially reducing the number of deaths from lung cancer by 20 percent. Finally, after decades of debate, the influential U.S. Preventative Task Force (USPTF) has issued guidelines for annual screening for lung cancer with low-dose computed tomography in adults aged 55 to 80 who have a 30 pack-year smoking history and currently smoke or have quit within the past 15 years.[3]

The Affordable Care Act now requires that all private insurers cover CT lung screening for those at high risk with no co-pay. In 2015, the Centers for Medicare & Medicaid Services, a federal agency within the U.S. Department of Health and Human Services, decided to provide CT lung screening coverage for Medicare beneficiaries at high risk, which estimates say number between three and four million people. Helping matters are the results of a cost-benefit analysis published last summer in the journal *American Health and Drug Benefits*. The study concluded that use of USPTF lung cancer screening recommendations in high-risk Medicare beneficiaries was cost-effective and that "Medicare should rapidly provide full national coverage for these exams."[4] These findings echo a 2012 study published in the journal *Health Affairs* that found low-dose CT lung cancer screening is cost-effective in high-risk traditionally insured people.[5]

Here's the bottom line: Screening in high-risk patients could save up to 30,000 people's lives each year. This is welcome and seriously overdue legislation. Wouldn't it be worth it if this were your parent, sibling, spouse, or other loved one? Or if it were you?

Here's what we know about lung cancer right now:

- Lung cancer may be lurking for decades before symptoms appear.
- Without screening, the disease will be too far advanced at the time of diagnosis to help a majority of lung cancer patients.

Given these two known facts, why would anyone still resist the idea that screening and early detection save lives?

In a perfect world, I'd love to see a lung cancer–screening program that embodies the following elements:

- A comprehensive lung cancer education program that informs those most at risk, as well as the public at large, of the most important risk factors.

- A nationwide campaign encouraging people to stop smoking and get a CT scan of their chest to detect the presence of any lung abnormalities.
- Smoking cessation and counseling programs to help nicotine addicts overcome this destructive habit.

If screening reveals an underlying abnormality—even if it turns out to be benign—it's critical to have a qualified medical professional review and explain the results, discuss all possible options, and educate you as to what the next steps might be.

The hope of screening advocates, myself included, is a simple one: to diagnose lung cancer in the earliest stages when the opportunity for a cure is greatest.

Lung Cancer Presentation

What do we mean by the term "clinical presentation"? Let me offer a simple explanation. "Clinical presentation" refers to the collection of disease-related signs and symptoms that eventually lead to the accurate diagnosis of a specific condition. As I've already noted, several times, early signs and symptoms are overlooked or simply don't exist, allowing lung cancer to go undetected for many years. And when signs and symptoms do surface, they are nonspecific and may appear at first glance to have little to do with the disease. This lack of specificity can often delay the correct diagnosis.

Lung cancer also is a true medical chameleon: It changes color quickly and doesn't always show up the same way. Tumor location and lymph node involvement, and secondary organ involvement are among the many factors influencing clinical presentation. There is also overlap between these groups. For example, a metastatic lung cancer patient might have symptoms from all the aforementioned categories or have only localized symptoms.[6]

Localized Lung Cancer Symptoms

Localized lung cancer means there's a tumor in the lung that may (or may not) have spread to local lymph nodes but hasn't spread further. For example, Stage II non–small cell lung cancer is defined as a "localized cancer." A cough is the number one localized lung cancer symptom, affecting more than 50 percent of patients. "New and persistent" is how doctors would label this cough both in nonsmokers and long-term former smokers like my patient Jack. In patients with a preexisting lung disease such as emphysema or chronic obstructive pulmonary disease (COPD), it's a change in the usual cough that precedes a lung cancer diagnosis.

Lung cancer patients may experience hemoptysis, a fancy way of saying "coughing up blood," which ranges from a few drops to a spewing stream of pure blood, the latter signaling a medical emergency. Pneumonia and other conditions trigger hemoptysis as well and also demand immediate medical attention. Unintentional weight loss, dyspnea (painful breathing), chest pain, and stridor—a strident, vibrating noise caused by an obstruction of the larynx—are also common symptoms.[7]

The Next Stage: Locally Advanced Lung Cancer

The shift from a "localized" lung cancer diagnosis to a "locally advanced" lung cancer may not sound like much, but it's actually a very big deal, as it signifies that cancer is no longer only in the lungs but has metastasized to structures in or adjacent to the lungs, or spread from regional lymph nodes. This is still considered "early-stage" disease, but it packs some nasty symptoms, including persistent hoarseness and/or difficulty swallowing. These symptoms could signify regional lymph node enlargement or indicate a lung tumor pressing against the esophagus. I have a patient who was legitimately shocked to learn that her nagging shoulder pain was actually an indication of locally advanced lung cancer. Facial swelling and overly prominent neck and chest veins may also indicate LALC.

Symptoms

Lung cancer is insidious, like all cancers. It can spread to virtually any organ, with the brain, liver, bones, and adrenal glands as the most common metastasis sites. Worst of all, early metastatic tumors may be asymptomatic, but as these secondary tumors grow, they can cause a lot of trouble.

Up to 20 percent of lung cancer patients may have paraneoplastic syndromes,[8] meaning that substances produced by the tumors, and not the tumors themselves, are causing signs and symptoms. Appetite change, constipation, weight loss, fever, exhaustion rashes, and edema all are paraneoplastic syndrome symptoms.

Diagnosing Lung Cancer

Obtaining an accurate diagnosis is one of the most challenging aspects of treating lung cancer. Diagnosis doesn't follow a straight path, and there isn't a single, universal test. Medical history, presenting complaints and symptoms, and results of a physical examination determine which tests are used. Patients need to know all their options.

Most people have an intuitive sense about their bodies. Although 5 percent of lung cancer patients present without symptoms, which doesn't mean they're asymptomatic but could mean that symptoms are not yet obvious, most people have an intuitive sense about their bodies and visit the doctor because they know something is not right. Typically, they're experiencing symptoms. Picture the diagnostic process as a big jigsaw puzzle. The first piece is always a detailed medical history, followed by a physical examination, during which the doctor gathers important information and considers and eliminates possible causes of your symptoms. "Do you smoke, or have you smoked, especially in the last 15 years? Have you been exposed to secondhand smoke or potential carcinogens?" "Have you experienced any problems with your lungs before?" "How long have been experiencing symptoms?" "Do you have a family history of cancer?" These are just some of the more common questions. This is why education regarding the importance of a screening CT of the chest is so important.

After taking a medical history, your doctor will conduct a physical exam and look for important lung cancer benchmarks such as a persistent cough, abnormal and/or labored breathing; swollen, tender glands or lymph nodes; bone pain or tenderness, back pain; muscle weakness or atrophy, rashes; changes in the lips or nails, and edema, specifically swelling in the hands, feet, and ankles. At the risk of sounding the alarm bells, any one of these symptoms could be a sign of a primary tumor. Of course, they may indicate nothing at all.

Common Tests

Laboratory testing and imaging are a standard part of any diagnostic workup. Patients often ask if there's a single definitive lung cancer test. A person's medical history, presenting symptoms, overall health, and exam findings all determine which test(s) a doctor orders. The following are the most common tests.

Sputum Cytology   Sputum is basically mucus, but if you want to get fancy, you can think of it as a thick saliva and fluid mixture that's secreted in the airways. Sputum cytology refers to a microscopic examination of mucus collected. Pathologists look for cancer cells under a microscope to look for cancer cells. Sputum cytology is a nerve-wracking test; a positive result usually means lung cancer, but a negative test doesn't rule out the possibility. Sputum cytology is positive in only 5 to 20 percent of lung cancer patients.[9]

Tumor Markers   Tumor markers are substances (biomarkers) in blood, urine, or tissue that are elevated only in people with cancer, or certain benign conditions. Carcinoembryonic antigen (CEA) is a tumor marker that's sometimes measured when lung cancer is suspected, but CEA is also elevated in the presence of other types of cancer.[10] Smokers also have abnormally high CEA levels, whether or not they have lung cancer, which only deepens the mystery. To date, there are no tumor markers for lung cancer that are sensitive to the presence of and specific for lung cancer.[11]

Imaging Tests   From chest X-rays to CT scans, imaging tests help determine whether further action is needed. Imaging tests also alert doctors to the presence of enlarged lymph nodes, an indication that the cancer may have spread outside the lung. Imaging helps, but the microscopic examination of lung tissue is the only way to conclusively rule out, or rule in, cancer.

Chest X-Rays   Chest X-ray is usually the first test ordered to identify any potential problem in the chest. It helps detect pleural effusion—the accumulation of fluid around the lung—and other cancer-correlated abnormalities such as enlarged lymph nodes, pneumonia, or obstructed airways. X-rays are ordered because they're easier to come by and comparatively inexpensive but are not great at picking up small lesions. Chest X-rays are no magical bullet, however. Sometimes they miss lung tumors; for example a small tumor hidden behind a rib, collarbone, or the breastbone might go unnoticed.

CT Scans   CT scans are the cornerstone of the diagnostic workup and help locate smaller tumors that evade X-ray detection. They collect three-dimensional images and thus help determine tumor size, shape, location, and the presence of enlarged lymph nodes. A spiral or helical CT scanner can examine the entire chest in less than 60 seconds, offering an even higher-quality image than older machines.

To Scan or Not to Scan

Hear ye, hear ye! I've been waiting for this, as have most of the doctors, surgeons, and health care practitioners who see lung cancer kill the many that could have been saved with early screenings. Lung cancer kills, so why be a victim? More people die of lung cancer each year (160,000) than the combined cancers of breast, colorectal, prostate, and ovarian. Currently, only 15 percent of all lung cancers are diagnosed early enough for cure.

In 2013, the U.S. Preventive Services Task Force issued guidelines recommending annual CT screening for current and former smokers aged 55 to 80 who smoked a pack a day for 30 years or 2 packs a day for 15 years (age 73 is when the majority of cases are diagnosed). The screening guidelines came about after the results of the National Cancer Institute–sponsored National Lung Screening Trial. According to findings published in the *New England Journal of Medicine,* low-dose CT screening reduced lung cancer mortality by 20 percent!

Low-dose CT screening can prevent as many as 20,000 deaths per year, and insurance companies will have to pay because it falls under the "preventive services" rubric. Advocacy groups and medical organizations like the American Cancer Society and the American Society of Clinical Oncology have already recommended lung cancer screening guidelines, but the U.S. Preventive Task Force recommendation is the final step in making chest CTs as common as mammograms and colonoscopies.

When lung cancers are found earlier, the five-year survival rate dramatically improves from 15 percent to more than 90 percent. Don't wait until you have symptoms because then it's too late.

Talk to your doctor to determine your personal risk of being affected.

Should I Get a CT Scan to Screen for Lung Cancer?

While some people can benefit immensely from a low-dose CT scan screening, it is not needed or helpful for everyone, and there are risks. Discussing your health history with your doctor will determine your best course of action. Ask questions. Contact your insurance provider to ensure CT screening is covered.

What Do the Results Mean?

A chest CT scan can reveal anything from a lung mass to emphysema, or nothing at all. However, what doctors term a "suspicious" result only means something is abnormal. This could indicate lung cancer or another serious condition. Even a "negative" result, meaning there were no abnormal findings on this CT scan, doesn't mean you're absolutely cancer free, or that you'll never get lung cancer. Knowing what to do next can be mindboggling. It pays to know your options! Additional procedures may be needed to determine what is abnormal. Your doctor can help review all available treatment options.

Find a physician who'll review the results of your CT scan. Formulating a plan if something is detected is just as important as scheduling surgery. Surgery is not always the best option but wouldn't you want to know if it is?

MRI Scans   Magnetic resonance imaging (MRI) scans also produce 3-D images and are used in lieu of an X-ray when there's a suspicion of lung cancer. An MRI is helpful for looking at an area that can't be properly interpreted from a CT scan, such as the diaphragm.

PET Scans   Positron emission tomography—PET scan for short—involves an intravenous injection of radioactive sugar molecules into the body before an image is taken. It's not as bad as it sounds because only a low amount of radiation is used. Some cancer cells grow and divide rapidly, devouring more sugar along the way. In a PET scan, cancer cells appear "brighter" than normal cells. PET scans help show these areas of activity, but recall, as previously said, that many cancers, including some lung tumors, grow slowly and are relatively inactive. Also, infections "eat sugar" as well, so the results need to be interpreted carefully with all aspects of the clinical scenario taken into account. PET scans are the best available imaging technology for determining whether cancer has spread to regional lymph nodes and for picking up distant metastases.

Next Steps: Tissue Diagnosis

Your doctor can only definitively diagnose cancer after examining a tissue sample under a microscope. Tissues samples are collected via a biopsy, which may only require a few cells (needle biopsy) or the resection of an entire lung mass. In some cases, minimally invasive surgery (MIS) allows us to resect the entire mass and have the tissue examined while the patient is still under anesthesia. The surgeon can then continue with further resection, if warranted by the specific situation. Every patient is different, and resecting a mass may be preferable to performing a needle biopsy if the patient is a good surgical candidate.

Bronchoscopy Bronchoscopy is procedure that looks inside the lungs' airways via a thin, lighted tube called a bronchoscope. Nowadays, the use of ultrasound (endobrachial ultrasound, or EBUS) or even computer technology (navigational bronchoscopy) can help find and sample lymph nodes or masses in the lung and chest. Bronchoscopy is usually performed on an outpatient basis.[12]

Mediastinoscopy Mediastinoscopy meets the real surgical procedure criteria and is performed under general anesthesia using an endoscope, a long, thin, flexible tube that's inserted through a small incision at the base of the neck or near the breastbone. It's a useful tool for both diagnosis and staging, which I discuss the next section of the chapter, because sampling the lymph nodes in the chest is critical for lung cancer staging. My patients appreciate the fact that, as a minimally invasive surgeon, I can sample most lymph nodes from the chest and therefore not leave a visible scar.

Transthoracic Needle Biopsy Transthoracic needle biopsy (TNB), or percutaneous needle aspiration, is performed via a hollow needle inserted through the chest and is generally used for tumors that may not be accessible with other techniques, usually if located near the surface. TNB collects lung tissue for testing and examination. It's often used to diagnose an irregular area of tissue in or around the lungs.

Core Needle Biopsy A core needle biopsy (CNB), also known as core biopsy or cutting needle biopsy, is a procedure in which a special needle is used to take a small cylinder-shaped (core) sample of tissue from a suspicious lump or mass. Along with aiding in diagnosis, CNB also helps doctors plan cancer surgery. The difference between CNB and TNB is needle size (core is larger) and CNB's increased risk of side effects such as bleeding or lung collapse. A CNB also obtains more tissue than TNB.

Video-Assisted Thoracoscopy Video-assisted thoracoscopy (VATS) is a technique I use frequently. By making a small incision in the chest, then inserting a tiny video camera, that projects pictures of the chest onto a large screen, the doctor has a close-up view during surgery. I perform single-incision procedures when I need to drain fluid or take tissue samples of the undersurface of the chest wall. Many times only local anesthesia with mild sedation is used. For more complicated procedures, a few more incisions need to be made, but there is no rib spreading, which allows for a quicker recovery and fewer days in the hospital. Seeking the opinion of a minimally invasive surgeon can help obtain an accurate diagnosis more easily and quickly.

Thoracotomy Thoracotomy is a major procedure that requires a large incision. The surgeon opens the chest and separates the rib cage, exposing the lungs. A hospital stay after thoracotomy can last anywhere from a week to five to ten days, depending on the patient's health and pain threshold. I use these incisions when the tumor is very large, but the goal is always smaller incisions for less pain and quicker recovery. Only 30 percent of chest surgeons use minimally invasive techniques, a statistic I'd like to see change.

The Big Show: Lung Cancer Staging

Once a definitive diagnosis is made, the next step is to determine how much cancer is in the body and how far it has advanced. Staging assesses the amount of cancer present in the tissues collected during one of the previously discussed diagnostic procedures. Imaging tests are useful also for lung cancer staging because they allow doctors to see the extent to which the cancer has grown and spread. Staging is broken into four categories.

Clinical staging determines how much cancer is present based on a physical examination, imaging tests, and biopsies.

Pathologic staging takes place only after a patient has undergone surgery to remove a tumor or explore the extent to which the cancer has spread. Pathologic staging results from both clinical staging and surgical results.

The third staging category, posttherapy or post-neoadjuvant therapy staging, is used to determine how much cancer remains after a patient is first treated with a systemic therapy (chemotherapy or hormone therapy) and/or a targeted therapy (radiation) before surgery or where no surgery is performed.

Restaging, which isn't always necessary, is performed to determine disease spread if there's a posttreatment disease recurrence. Restaging is helpful to determine the best of course of treatment.

Location and amount are central to lung cancer staging. Patients frequently question me about the need for staging. First of all, the stage—the point to which your cancer has progressed—often tells your doctor whether additional tests may be needed. Stage I lung cancer, where the tumor is small, limited to the lung, and hasn't spread to the lymph nodes, requires a much different treatment algorithm than Stage IV lung cancer, in which cancer has spread beyond the lung to distant sites.

Lung cancer patients who meet specific stage group criteria have a similar prognosis, although many factors, which I'll discuss at length in later chapters, can and do affect disease course and outcome. Lung cancer treatment, like everything else in medicine, isn't an exact science. Some people recover beyond what was expected, while others don't reach the minimally expected recovery.

Staging figures prominently in a doctor's assessment of a patient's prognosis (the anticipated disease course and outcome). Without staging, your doctor couldn't possibly devise an appropriate treatment plan. This last point is critical because as I've stated before many times, lung cancer may not always be curable, but it's always *treatable*.

Staging allows doctors to compare treatment paradigms and plan research. Also, it's not uncommon to stage lung cancer more than once. The first, or "clinical stage," is done before treatment. The second, or "pathologic stage," is performed after treatment and is considered a more precise measure of disease metastasis.

Lung cancer staging guidelines are under the aegis of the American Joint Committee on Cancer and the Union for International Cancer Control. In this system, the letters T, N, and M indicate a different cancer growth area and, based on the result, your doctor will assign a numerical score to each letter. However, not all cancers are rated with this system.

T = Tumor

"T" is the primary tumor rating, defining such critical pieces of information as size, location, and local invasion. This is obviously important because an untreated primary tumor can grow and spread quickly.

It can also grow through the tissue where it started, which is known as "tumor extension." This is letting the genie out of the proverbial bottle. These tumors can easily invade other neighboring structures. TX refers to a primary tumor that's too small to be evaluated. T0 indicates no evidence of a primary tumor. This refers to an early primary tumor that hasn't metastasized to the neighboring tissue. This cancer is only found in the top layers of cells lining the air passages.

T1 through T4 refer to the size and extent of the primary tumor:

- T1 indicates a tumor is no larger than 3 centimeters and slightly less than 1¼ centimeters in diameter. If the tumor is 2 centimeters or less across, it is called T1a. If the tumor is larger than 2 centimeters but not larger than 3 centimeters in diameter, it is classified as T1b. T2 tumors have spread into the visceral pleura, the membrane that surrounds the lungs.
- T2 tumors partially block the airways but haven't caused a pneumothorax or pneumonia. If a T2 tumor is 5 centimeters or less across, it is called T2a. If the tumor is larger than 5 centimeters across (but not larger than 7 centimeters), it is called T2b.
- A T3 tumor is greater than 7 centimeters across, has entered the chest wall, the breathing muscle that separates the chest from the abdomen (diaphragm), the membranes surrounding the space between the two lungs (mediastinal pleura), or membranes of the sac surrounding the heart (parietal pericardium). It has grown into a main bronchus and is closer than 2 centimeters (about three-quarters of an inch) to the carina (where the main brochi divides), but it does not involve the carina itself. It has grown into the airways enough to cause an entire lung to collapse or to cause pneumonia in the entire lung. Two or more separate tumor nodules are present in the same lobe of a lung.
- T4 is a tumor that's not classified by size (T4s can be of any size) but by whether it has spread to the structures of the mediastinum or backbone. T4 is an inoperable tumor even with minimally invasive surgery and is most often associated with lung and/or heart malignancies.[13]

N = Nodes

"N" indicates regional lymph node involvement. It reflects the extent to which cancer has spread to adjacent lymph nodes. Lung cancer cells can invade lymph vessels and travel to lymph nodes. Once there, they multiply and form new tumors. There are 14 different locations, or stations, in the chest where lymph nodes are found. They are categorized by anatomic location. However, lung cancer patients should be concerned with only five of these.

- Hilar lymph nodes are located at the site of entrance or exit of blood vessels and bronchi associated with the lungs.
- Mediastinal lymph nodes are found in the mediastinum, the space between the lungs. These nodes are classified according to location and their relation to the trachea esophagus, and aorta.
- Supraclavicular lymph nodes sit just above the clavicle.
- Ipsilateral lymph nodes (ipsilateral means situated on or affecting the same side) are found on the same side of the body as the tumor.
- Contralateral lymph nodes are on the other side of the chest, away from the tumor.

Cancer in lymph nodes other than the hilar, mediastinal, and supraclavicular lymph nodes are evidence of distant metastases.

Cancer in adjacent lymph nodes and the number and/or region of cancer nodes are the criteria on which doctors base "N" scores. A "NX" score means that the lymph nodes can't be assessed.

An "N" designation indicates lymph node cancer involvement. "N0" means that no cancer was found in any regional lymph nodes. N1 indicates cancer has moved to the ipsilateral hilar lymph nodes; N2 is cancer in the mediastinal or subcarinal lymph nodes; and N3 is a metastasis in contralateral mediastinal, contralateral hilar, ipsilateral or contralateral scalene, or supraclavicular lymph node(s).[14]

M = Metastasis

"M" is all about the disease spread. The M designation reflects the extent to which the cancer has metastasized to distant sites. Generally, physicians try to establish the M factor early in the staging process because the presence of a distant tumor indicates that a person has progressed (or should I say "regressed") to Stage IV. An "M0" score means there's no cancer lurking about at distant sites. This happens with occult lung cancer, where tumor cells show up in the sputum or bronchial washings (a rinse solution obtained during bronchoscopy), but imaging studies or direct examination with a bronchoscope don't detect a primary tumor. M1 indicates distant metastasis.

If a distant metastasis is found and Stage IV lung cancer has been diagnosed, no further staging procedures are needed.[15] M1a is a separate tumor nodule(s) in an opposite lobe from the primary metastasis, a tumor with pleural nodules or malignant pleural (or pericardial) effusion. M1b is a distant metastasis in organs outside the chest.

Lung Cancer Stages

Using the universal American Joint Committee on Cancer (AJCC) and Union for International Cancer Control (UICC) classification systems, we can break non–small cell and small cell lung cancers into the following stages.

Non–Small Cell Lung Cancer

Non–small cell lung cancer is divided into the following four stages.

Stage I   Stage I is a malignant tumor that hasn't moved beyond the primary, or original, tumor site or invaded regional lymph nodes. Stage IA tumors are small (less than three centimeters) but IB tumors are larger. Stage I tumors are considered curable with surgery.

Stage II   Stage II NSCLC indicates a primary tumor that's spread to the ipsilateral hilar lymph nodes. As in Stage I, a Stage IIA tumor is three centimeters or less in diameter; Stage IIB is greater than three centimeters. As an example, a Stage IIB tumor has no hilar lymph node involvement and surgeons consider it curable, although the chance of recurrence is higher than for Stage I patients.

Stage III   The stakes rise with Stage III cancer. As a more complex disease, there's general medical consensus that Stage IIIA and IIIB disease can't be treated the same way. A Stage IIIA tumor has invaded the chest wall, diaphragm, and the pleura and also indicates ipsilateral hilar or mediastinal lymph node involvement. Still, these tumors are potentially operable. Stage IIIB disease includes any size tumor that has invaded any of the mediastinum, carina, or spine vital structures, with or without regional lymph node involvement. However, Stage IIIB patients aren't good surgical candidates because their cancerous tissue has spread well beyond the primary tumor site.

Stage IV   Stage IV indicates a distant metastasis, meaning the disease has spread beyond the regional lymph nodes and primary tumor site.[16] This is advanced-stage disease, and treatment focuses on palliation (efforts to relieve pain and symptoms), as opposed to cure.

Small Cell Lung Cancer

The AJCC and CUICC classification and staging systems apply both to SCLC and NSCLC because the size of the tumor and/or degree of lymph node involvement between these two cancers are similar. The two systems allow us to assess patient prognosis and determine treatment options. A crucial difference between the two types of cancer, however, is that small lung cell cancers grow and metastasize quickly, a point I discussed earlier.[17]

SCLC patients are staged with limited or extensive disease based on the amount of cancer in the chest. "Limited stage SCLC" is a tumor confined to one lung, the mediastinum, and/or the regional lymph nodes. For the 30 percent of people who have limited-stage SCLC at time of diagnosis, disease treatment involves a combination of chemotherapy and thoracic radiation. For some reason, SCLC doesn't respond well to targeted therapies, and attempts have yielded disappointing results, although a recent clinical trial of untreated extensive-stage SCLC patients with the drug sunitinib showed a "modest but significant improvement in . . . survival from 2.1 months with placebo to 3.7 months."[18] I discuss treatment at greater length in the next chapter. Limited stage corresponds to Stages I through IIIB, according to the AJCC staging algorithm.

Extensive, or widespread, SCLC, on the other hand, means the cancer has spread beyond the primary tumor. In fact, an estimated 70 percent of SCLC patients have extensive stage disease at the time of diagnosis.

Going Forward

Common sense and science are two requirements for practicing medicine. My patients are up to speed on the latest diagnostic and treatment techniques. Accurately diagnosing and staging lung cancer is the key to survival. It doesn't have to involve many stressful tests or trips to the hospital. You have to evaluate and communicate test findings in a way that's understandable for a majority of people. It's gratifying when people leave my office with a clear picture of the road ahead. My goal is to lessen any unnecessary stress they're experiencing.

Pulling It All Together

If you have any symptoms that possibly indicate lung cancer, especially if you're part of a high-risk demographic, your doctor will first conduct a physical examination. Depending on the findings, more tests may be ordered, including, but not limited to, blood work, a CT scan, and X-rays. If the tests come back positive or indicate something suspicious, your doctor will order or perform an additional biopsy using any number of techniques, including a bronchoscopy, a fine needle biopsy, thoracentesis, or VATS (video-assisted thoracic surgery). Some lung cancers may also be tested for abnormal proteins (biomarkers) or DNA mutations.

Once a lung cancer diagnosis is made, it's important to determine tumor size, spread (if any), and location, which is called staging. Staging is critical for determining the best course of treatment. There are four stages of lung cancer treatment. In general, Stage I and II tumors are smaller and haven't spread too much, whereas Stage III and IV tumors are bigger and have spread beyond the primary tumor site. Lung cancer is typically categorized as either limited or extensive.

Step III
Know Your Options

CHAPTER 5

Treating Lung Cancer

Takeaways

- Lung cancer treatment includes surgery, chemotherapy, radiation, targeted drug therapy, immunotherapy, and palliative care. Surgery and radiation therapy treat localized lung cancer; chemotherapy, on the other hand, is a systemic therapy that kills cancer cells throughout the body.
- There's no one ideal lung cancer treatment; it typically involves a number of therapies and depends on the type of lung cancer, disease progression, ancillary/secondary illnesses (comorbidity), overall health, personality style, and psychological makeup.
- Lung cancer disappears in a small percentage of patients without standard medical intervention. Such "radical remissions" are rare occurrences, however, and shouldn't be counted on as a viable treatment option.

Introduction

In the 17 years that I've been practicing medicine, lung cancer information and treatment options have changed for the better. Although chemotherapy, radiation therapy, and surgery remain the gold standard, research has paved the way for new advances, including ways to treat and even cure lung cancer. Improved radiation techniques and Food and Drug Administration (FDA) approval of immunotherapy (a new treatment that targets a specific feature of the cancer and activates the immune system against the disease) are now being used alone or in combination, depending on lung cancer type and disease stage. My goal is to present an overview of each therapy and its application in treating lung cancer.

There are 7,856 terms in the National Cancer Institute's *Dictionary of Cancer Terms*. I can safely say there isn't a doctor on the planet capable of defining them all. Included in this extensive list are a number of treatment options, which change almost daily as we learn more and more about lung cancer and new treatments become part of clinical practice. Like all aspects of cancer care, treatment has its own expressions and idioms. Early on, I define and explain a number of terms common to treatment language. If a doctor or other health care professionals use a term that causes your eyes to glaze over or talks over your head, ask for an explanation. There are no dumb questions; we're talking about your health. If a doctor or other health care professional dismisses your concerns, find another provider. I answer questions every day. It's my job. Hopefully, you only do this once. Any doctor worth his or her reputation should have no problem answering the same questions again and again.

Talking the Talk: The Language of Lung Cancer Treatment

Response to Therapy

"Response to therapy" means just what the term implies: the patient responds to a given treatment. A "complete response" (and the outcome we all hope for, of course) is the disappearance of all cancer symptoms after treatment. However, this doesn't imply a cure because cancer is a tricky disease and there can be residual cancer cells that go undetected, even in someone who's been declared "in remission" or "cancer free," explaining why patients are monitored for years after treatment.

On the flipside of the same coin, a "partial or incomplete remission" is all about tumor size shrinkage and/or disappearance of cancer. Response to therapy is about slowing down disease progression. If your doctor says you're "responding" to therapy, be happy, but don't announce to the world that you're cancer free, either. Please understand that a "response" to therapy is about treatment, but it doesn't imply cure. Many cancers respond well to treatment but still hang around after the sheriff skips town.

"Progressive disease" means the cancer is continuing unabated. If you're receiving treatment and the disease is still marching forward, discuss stopping the treatment with your doctor.

All of the preceding expressions are considered "endpoints." But an endpoint also refers to an outcome doctors or researchers are trying to measure with a clinical trial. All peer-reviewed medical literature reporting the results of clinical trials will refer to the results in terms of "measured endpoints." For our purposes, we should focus on the "endpoint" as it relates to treatment effectiveness, also called "efficacy endpoints." Doctors also use the term when reviewing expected treatment benefits with patients or discussing how a patient is responding to treatment.

Common Treatment Descriptions

- First-line therapy—The first therapy used to treat a disease. In the case of lung cancer, it could be part of a set of treatments such as surgery followed by chemotherapy and radiation.
- Second-line therapy—Doctors turn to this therapy if the initial treatment doesn't work, that is, if there's evidence of disease progression after the first round of therapy is completed.
- Treatment-naive—These are first-timers, or patients who've never undergone treatment for a specific illness.
- Curative intent—Treatment designed to cure disease.[1]
- Multimodality therapy—Also referred to as "combination therapy," this indicates two or more treatment modalities used together.
- Adjuvant treatment—Treatment that follows the primary therapy to increase the likelihood of a cure. Chemotherapy and radiation are adjuvant lung cancer therapies when administered after surgery.
- Neoadjuvant therapy—Also known as "induction therapy," neoadjuvant therapy is given before primary therapy to increase the chance of a cure. For example, chemotherapy and radiation before surgery are neoadjuvant therapies. However, when used after surgery, they are considered adjuvant therapies.[2]
- Palliative therapy—This is all about symptom alleviation after a diagnosis of late-stage (Stage IV) cancer. Palliative therapy isn't curative and doesn't change disease course, but it can significantly improve the quality of life, which is why it's an integral part of my medical practice.[3]

Treatment Effectiveness: How to Decide

"What's the best lung cancer treatment?" an elderly patient asked me not too long ago.

As with most things, there is no one-size-fits-all answer. Patients should consider a number of options before deciding on treatment, including clinical trials if the diagnosis is grave or seems to warrant such an intervention. Clinical trials are research studies that test the safety and efficacy of new treatment approaches and try to determine see whether a given new approach works better than standard treatment. Clinical trials typically include a new drug, a new combination of standard treatments, or new doses of current therapies.

Treatment Overview

Lung cancer treatment falls into four basic categories: surgery, radiation therapy, chemotherapy, and targeted therapy. I describe each treatment in greater detail in the next sections, followed by an outline of common treatment plans by cancer type and stage. Type and cancer stage, possible side effects, as well as the patient's preferences, overall health, and insurance, all play a role in determining treatment plans. My best advice is that you familiarize yourself with all possible treatment options, ask questions, and discuss with your doctor the goals of each treatment and what you can expect while undergoing treatment.

No discussion of treatment effectiveness would be complete without a caveat about numbers. Clinical trial numbers mean a lot. How else are scientists to compare treatments? When it comes time for you, the cancer patient, to make a treatment decision, don't think the numbers necessarily correlate with your own specific chance of responding to a given therapy. Maybe you read or your doctor told you that a certain drug has a 40 percent "response rate." What this means, simply, is that 40 percent of people treated with this drug responded to it. It doesn't mean you also have a 40 percent chance of responding to this drug. Many factors effect response rate. Your cancer's genetic makeup, your immune response, the presence of other illnesses (comorbidity), age, gender, and stress all may contribute to your response rate to a given therapy.

Use statistics as a barometer, but don't overestimate the impact of treatment trial numbers on your personal situation. Numbers mean something, but they don't measure your unique genetic makeup, biology, and personality style, and thus they can't gauge your personal response to any given treatment. The correlation I'd draw is with fertility and age. Statistically, fertility rates drop significantly after a woman reaches age 35. However, many women over 35, and even 40, get pregnant and go on to deliver perfectly healthy babies. Similarly, no one can put a number on the outcome of your disease. Lung cancer survival stats can be discouraging, to say the least. On the other hand, millions survive without any recurrence of their cancer. Why not you?

Radical Remissions: Can You Defy the Odds?

Their stories are the stuff of legend: People diagnosed with late-stage cancer only to have their disease disappear a short time later—all without treatment. Such "spontaneous remissions" are rare. How is it someone given just two years to live can survive another 40? What causes a large aggressive tumor, such as malignant melanoma (which can spread to the lungs if left untreated), to just disappear off the map?

It's really impossible to quantify the occurrence of spontaneous remissions—numbers range from 1 in 60,000 to 1 in 100,000 patients—since they're frequently based on anecdotal accounts. All too often, when fully studied, it is shown that there was never a cancer at all, so there was no "remission." But real cases of spontaneous remission do exist.[4] These people, sometimes called "exceptional patients," have begun to attract the attention of researchers who are interested in what, if anything, they're doing to heal themselves of incurable diseases or to improve their chances of being cured.

There's been some research into the idea of spontaneous or radical remissions. In 1993, the Institute of Noetic Sciences published *Spontaneous Remissions: An Annotated Bibliography*, which cataloged all existing medical (peer-reviewed) literature on the subject. It included references to cancer and a wide range of illnesses—from ulcers to injuries caused by gunshots—and includes the largest existing database of spontaneous remission in the world, with more than 3,500 references from more than 800 journals in 20 languages.[5]

Although any number of factors may contribute to spontaneous remission, the real clues originate our own immune system.

In one celebrated case, a man diagnosed with late-stage malignant melanoma, which had spread to his lungs, developed white rings around his skin lesions following a month-long regimen of healthy living, leading researchers to theorize that the patient's immune system was mobilizing against melanocytes, pigmented cells in the skin that are the source of this form of skin cancer. Although most doctors say it's impossible to know just what causes the immune system to kick suddenly into action and induce a remission in any individual patient, this case underscores questions that researchers would like to answer: Did this patient's month of hiking, healthy eating, and meditating inadvertently supercharge his immune system? Did another, as-of-yet unidentified factor make his lung tumor mysteriously disappear?[6]

In her celebrated book, *Radical Remission: Surviving Cancer Against All Odds*, Kelly Turner, PhD, analyzed more than 1,000 cases of spontaneous remission. Dr. Turner, who favors the term "radical remission" because typically there is nothing spontaneous about these unusual cures, feels that most patients who experience a reversal of their cancer are actively doing something to facilitate healing.[7]

Dr. Turner has identified more than 75 healing factors that these patients used to help heal themselves, including diet change, taking charge of their health, using medicinal herbs and supplements, releasing bottled-up emotions and incorporating positive psychology, setting up and utilizing social supports, strengthening their spirituality, and recognizing reasons to live.

Not surprisingly, the most critical healing factors involved a combination of body, mind, and spirit interventions. Dr. Turner is quick to point out that she's promoting a program to cure cancer. As she told *Medscape Medical News*, "[This isn't a] '9 steps to curing cancer' sort of thing . . . you can't do that. This is not a 9-step program for getting well. These are just 9 factors that most of the survivors had in common."[8]

Dr. Turner's research focused on three categories of cancer patients: those who healed from their disease without the use of any standard/conventional medicine; those who were treated with standard therapy and, when it failed to work, tried other treatments that did help; and those who used conventional and alternative medicine at the same time to overcome a very serious prognosis, such as advanced lung or pancreatic cancer.

In one case, the tumors of a patient with Stage III non–small cell lung cancer had shrunk to almost undetectable levels and weren't causing any trouble. This patient never received any standard treatment for his lung cancer but used a form of energy work and kept asking his doctors for "six more months" before beginning chemotherapy. Six months turned into a year, and now it's been five years.

In all my years practicing medicine, I've never personally encountered a case of spontaneous/radical remission. Although I don't want to give false hope or create unrealistic expectations, there are people whose cancer disappears. We should talk about them. If we ignore—or worse, dismiss—the incidence of spontaneous remission, we could be missing out on an opportunity to learn how cancer behaves and about the healing process. We can learn a lot by studying anomalies.

Chemotherapy

Cancer and chemotherapy are two of the most closely associated words in the English language—flip sides of the same coin. Recent medical advances notwithstanding, if you have anything beyond early-stage cancer, chances are that you'll soon be on a first-name basis with chemotherapy. But what is it anyway? In simple terms, chemotherapy is the use of medicine to treat cancer. Chemotherapy drugs kill cancer cells.

Some chemotherapy drugs interfere with cancer cell division; others wreck havoc with a cell's DNA, preventing self-repair, which leads to cell death, or apoptosis. All chemotherapy drugs adhere to a single, fundamental principle: they target mechanisms active in rapidly growing and dividing cells. Whether in combination or individually to increase treatment response, chemotherapy drugs are always given with the same goal in mind. The problem with chemotherapy drugs—and chemotherapy in general—is that the drugs work systemically and can't distinguish between normal cells and cancer cells, which accounts for the unpleasant side effects you've probably heard about, or may have even experienced.

Why Is Chemotherapy Used?

Given the terrible side effects, patients frequently ask me why chemotherapy seems to be the default choice to deal with cancer. Because chemotherapy is "systemic" therapy (i.e., it affects the entire system, or body), unlike radiation, it's incorporated when it is certain the cancer has spread beyond its initial site or it appears that micrometastasis (i.e., cancer cells too small to show up in tests) are present. Chemotherapy is an effective cancer therapy because it shrinks tumors, prolongs life by slowing cancer growth, and prevents cancer spread. Even when chemotherapy doesn't lead to cure—it never cures late-stage cancer—it can relieve symptoms and extend life.

How Do We Administer Chemotherapy Drugs?

Chemotherapy most often is given through a needle right into your bloodstream. Chemotherapy drugs can also be taken orally. Treatment can last a few hours, or can be spread over several days via a continuous drip. Whatever the specific schedule, most chemotherapy drugs need time to take effect. And the breaks between treatments also give normal cells time to recover.

Chemotherapy Side Effects

Chemotherapy side effects are a real concern for my patients. Side effect severity varies, however. No two people react the same to a given treatment. Dosage, your body's reaction, and even the drug itself affect the intensity and frequency of side effects. Chemotherapy doesn't discriminate—the drugs don't kill cancer cells alone. Chemotherapy damages rapidly growing and dividing tissue, such as that lining the inside of the throat and mouth. This helps explain why many cancer patients are susceptible to mouth sores and taste changes. Myelosuppression, a condition in which bone marrow activity decreases, resulting in fewer red blood cells, white blood cells, and platelets (severe myelosuppression is called myeloablation), is another chemotherapy side effect. Myelosuppression also is a common "dose-limiting side effect," meaning the treatment or individual drug side effects are serious enough to prevent a dose or level increase of that treatment. This category of side effects may prompt your doctor to lower the dose or prolong treatment intervals. In extreme cases, the drug in question may need to be eliminated altogether.

Cancer cells grow and divide quickly. Chemotherapy drugs impair cancer cell growth and division. Growing hair also involves rapid cell division, explaining how and why 70 percent of chemotherapy drugs damage hair follicles, causing partial or complete hair loss.

Chemotherapy's Most Common Side Effects

The following are the 11 most common side effects associated with chemotherapeutic drugs commonly used to treat lung cancer. Chemotherapy doesn't affect two people the same way. I've seen patients sail through chemotherapy with few, or even no, side effects. On the other hand, some patients turn sick and miserable after a single dose. Every person is different, and I tell my patients that they can always stop. However, if they don't do anything, the cancer wins.

1. Constipation
2. Diarrhea
3. Fatigue
4. Hair loss (alopecia)
5. Appetite loss/taste changes
6. Fatigue and memory loss
7. Painful mouth sores, dry mouth, and taste changes
8. Myelosuppression, including anemia (low red blood cell count), neutropenia (low white blood cell count), and thrombocytopenia (low platelet count)
9. Nausea and vomiting
10. Peripheral neuropathy (numbness, tingling, and pain in the hands and feet that is similar to what diabetes patients experience)
11. Edema (swelling)

Radiation Therapy

What Is Radiation Therapy?

Radiation therapy, or radiotherapy, is a common lung cancer treatment. It targets concentrated energy beams at cancer cells, damaging their genetic blueprint, stopping cell division, and blocking new cancer cell formation. Healthy cells usually revive, but the treatment destroys cancer cells. Stripped of their ability to self-repair, the cells die. Radiation doses administered during cancer treatment are several thousand times stronger than X-ray radiation exposure. Like chemotherapy, radiation doesn't discriminate. It kills both good and bad cells. Modern technology has sharpened radiation's focus, allowing for a more targeted treatment of cancer cells.

Why Do We Use Radiation Therapy?

Radiation therapy is "local," meaning it only affects cells in the treatment area. In this way, it differs radically from chemotherapy, a systemic treatment that can't tell the difference between good and bad cells. Radiotherapy is a lung cancer "adjuvant therapy," meaning it's administered in combination with surgery and/or chemotherapy.[9] Before surgery, radiation is used to shrink tumor size, which aids in resection, eases cancer-associated pain, increases a patient's responsiveness to treatment, and, hopefully, kills lingering postsurgical cancer cells. Radiotherapy also relieves disease-related symptoms and prolongs life if a cure is unlikely.[10]

How Is Radiation Therapy Given?

There are three ways to administer radiation therapy: externally, internally, or systemically (radiation is sometimes given in more than one way during a specific treatment). As the name implies, *external beam radiation*, or external beam therapy, is applied outside the body using a machine called a linear accelerator. It's the most widely used radiation therapy type and is used to treat large surfaces and more than one area of the body. External beam radiation can be delivered in a number of ways. *Three-dimensional conformal radiation therapy (3D-CRT)* maps the tumor location using imaging techniques. The radiation beams matching the tumor shape are delivered in several directions. This is a highly precise treatment designed to minimize radiation damage to surrounding tissues while simultaneously increasing the radiation dose. A significant drawback of 3D-CRT is that imaging tests don't always allow the radiologist to see the full extent of the disease, meaning that some parts of the tumor won't get treated.[11]

Intensity modulated radiation therapy (IMRT) is an advanced form of external radiation therapy. As with 3D-CRT, radiologists map a three-dimensional image. This therapy also delivers radiation beams in several directions, but beam strength can also be adjusted, sparing the surrounding normal tissues.[12]

Volumetric modulated arc therapy (VMAT) is an IMRT variation that rotates once around the body, delivering short, precise radiation doses in a treatment that lasts just a few minutes. VMAT is convenient for the patients, but it's not yet known if it's as effective or more effective than regular IMRT. Because IMRT and VMAT use higher total doses of radiation than other modalities, patients may be at a slightly increased risk of treatment-related secondary cancers.[13]

Image-guided radiation therapy (IGRT) is a scanner technology that enables a surgeon, just before radiation treatment, to deliver even more precise radiation doses by getting pictures of the tumor. The result is fewer side effects.[14]

Intensity modulated proton therapy (IMPT) is an IMRT that uses proton beams instead of photon beams, allowing for more radiation delivery to the tumor site. There's also evidence suggesting that IMPT improves cancer outcomes. IMPT is often used for tumors near critical body structures, such as the eye, brain, and spine.

Other radiation therapies include the following:

- *Stereotactic radiosurgery (SRS) and fractionated stereotactic radiotherapy*, which deliver a large, precise radiation dose to a small, well-defined tumor.
- *Stereotactic body radiation therapy (SBRT)*, a technique used to treat for tumors in other body parts.
- *Intraoperative radiation therapy (IORT)*, radiation given during surgery for cancers deep inside the body (normal tissues can be moved aside during surgery, exposing the cancer).
- *Electromagnetic-guided radiation therapy*, sometimes known as 4-D therapy because it includes a radiation planning formula using electromagnetic implants or "transponders" to send out radio waves that tell radiation therapy machines where to aim.

Internal Radiation

Internal beam radiation brachytherapy is internal radiation treatment. High dose rate (HDR) brachytherapy delivers radiation from implants placed close to, or inside the tumor(s). Because cancer can, and often does, affect organs and other essential structures, radiation treatment is given with the idea of minimizing serious side effects. HDR brachytherapy offers the maximum radiation dose, while minimizing exposure to surrounding healthy tissue. This pinpoint focus inside tumors makes HDR brachytherapy a potentially beneficial lung cancer treatment.[15]

Successful radiotherapy requires planning. Radiation oncologists—physicians specializing in radiation treatment of cancer—map out the dose and treatment schedule. Radiotherapy is a gradual process, administered in small doses (fractionating) over a period of two to eight weeks, allowing normal cells enough down time to recover, while minimizing damage to healthy tissues. Tumor size and location, adjuvant treatments, the presence of other metastases, and the patient's general health and state of mind all affect radiation dose and schedule.[16]

A surprising fact about radiotherapy is that the first treatment isn't a treatment at all. Before radiation therapy, patients go through a "simulation," which is a radiation therapy planning session. Because positioning is critical with radiation therapy, your doctor will order a CT scan of the treatment region before radiation, which creates a roadmap for your doctor to design a treatment plan. Simulation allows doctors to map the radiotherapy target area, or "port," to get the biggest bang for the buck while limiting exposure to healthy tissues.[17]

Radiation Therapy Side Effects

You'd expect anything strong enough to kill cancer cells to have a number of unpleasant and often serious side effects. Fractional radiation dosing produces fewer and less adverse side effects, but there's no getting away scot-free either. Fortunately, the majority of radiation side effects are local, meaning they occur only in the treatment field. Cough, chest discomfort, fatigue, shortness of breath, hair loss, appetite loss, skin and mouth problems, sore throat, and even impaired cognitive functioning are the most common treatment side effects. Skin is especially susceptible to radiotherapy side effects, and the treated area may feel noticeably sore, dry, or itchy and darken or redden.[18] More serious radiation side effects and complications include esophagitis (inflammation of the esophagus), sore throat, pain, heartburn, and difficulty swallowing.[19]

Radiation pneumonitis, a condition that results from damage to the lining of the airways and air sacs, is a treatment side effect affecting 2 to 9 percent of lung cancer patients who undergo radiotherapy.[20] Radiation pneumonitis symptoms mimic those associated with pneumonia, including cough, low fever, shortness of breath, and/or pain associated with breathing. Women, interestingly, are slightly more prone to developing this complication than men.[21] Not surprisingly, smoking increases pneumonitis risk for both men and women.[22] Prednisone (Cortan, Deltasone), azathioprine (Imuran), and cyclosporine (Neoral, Sandimmune) are used to treat radiation pneumonitis.[23]

Amifostine (Ethyol) is a radioprotectant and, as the classification implies, a drug that protects healthy tissues from radiotherapy damage without interfering with treatment effectiveness. Amifostine also protects the kidneys from harmful effects caused by cisplatin, a common chemotherapy drug.

Proton Therapy

Between 15 and 20 percent of lung cancer patients have tumors that can be treated surgically or by surgery combined with other therapies. Another 30 to 50 percent have locally advanced tumors that require a combined treatment regimen that includes radiation and/or chemotherapy.[24] The lungs' proximity to other organs makes delivering a proper or adequate radiation dose challenging. Enter proton therapy, a recently developed treatment that uses an advanced image guidance system to deliver targeted, powerful radiation dosages, sparing critical nearby structures. Protons are positively charged particles found in the nucleus of an atom. Proton therapy enables a doctor to treat the tumor with a higher dose of radiation, resulting in better local control of the disease, higher survival rates, and improved quality of life. Proton therapy may also benefit patients with recurrent lung cancer and those who've already received radiation therapy. In this case, pencil beam limits or eliminates radiation to these sensitive areas.[25,26]

Surgical Procedures

Today, lung cancer surgery is at a crossroads. New, cutting-edge, minimally invasive techniques are revolutionizing the field of thoracic surgery, offering patients lower infection and complication rates and shorter hospitals stays, while lessening the need for pain medications. Yet almost 50 percent of lung cancer patients still undergo open-chest surgery, even though minimally invasive lung surgery offers a number of benefits. To me, this is an unconscionable discrepancy, considering the risks from more invasive procedures. In pancreatic surgery, as an example, minimally invasive techniques cause infection in 1 percent of cases, whereas open procedures cause infection in 12 to 15 percent of cases.[27] Imagine a pill that reduced the incidence of postsurgical infection. Everyone would be using it.

A study published in the *Journal of the American Medical Association* implied that increasing the number of minimally invasive procedures offered in hospitals favoring open procedures would result in 4,300 fewer complications, nearly 170,000 fewer hospital days, and $337 million in annual savings nationwide. Fewer complications, as an example, would save an average of $2,844 per patient undergoing a lobectomy. Factoring in other variables, such as reduced length of stay, increased per patient savings to $6,209.[28,29]

For hospitals, surgery is a big-ticket item, and surgical admissions constitute 50 percent of admissions at the country's biggest hospitals. Shorter stays equate to fewer dollars. At some hospitals, volume is the basis for surgical compensation, so physicians don't refer patients to minimally invasive surgeons. I know doctors who've deliberately steered patients away from minimally invasive surgery, even calling it "dangerous" and "experimental." "My other doctor never presented minimally invasive surgery as an option," a number of patients have told me.

In a perfect world, we'd only place patients in situations that yield the best outcome. If a lung cancer patient is a minimally invasive surgical candidate, why is he or she going to a doctor who only performs open procedures?

All of this underscores the need to have the right information and to ask the right questions. Bottom line: Without the large incision used in traditional lung surgery, minimally invasive surgery means faster healing, shorter hospital stays, reduced costs, less postoperative pain, and minimal scarring and blood loss. What could be wrong with that?

When Is Surgery Used?

Cure or symptom alleviation is surgery's goal. Surgery is considered a cure for early-stage or localized lung cancer. Patients with early-stage lung cancer should find a thoracic surgeon experienced in lung cancer surgery and who's trained in minimally invasive surgical techniques.

Ideally, lung resection surgery should be performed using minimally invasive techniques, including video-assisted thoracic surgery (VATS), which involves the insertion of a tiny camera, or thoracoscope, through a small incision, allowing a surgeon to view and examine the chest cavity. Unfortunately, thoracotomy, a more invasive technique that involves a longer, more painful recovery, is still the procedure of choice for the majority of surgeons worldwide. Specially designed instruments help the surgeon remove tissue, while 3D imaging technology, a fairly recent development, assists with visualization, just like robotic surgery, except that the surgeon is physically at the operating table.

Like VATS, robotic thoracic surgery is another minimally invasive procedure that gives a surgeon access inside the chest cavity through small incisions. The robotic system provides excellent visualization (using 3D technology) with the surgeon at a console in the same room.

When a mass needs to be resected or cancer is found, procedures using VATS or a robot-assisted technique may include:

- A *wedge resection* is a removal of the tumor itself and surrounding tissue. A wedge resection is performed on growths near the lung's surface if your surgeon feels a more extensive procedure wouldn't be well tolerated.
- A *segmentectomy* or *bronchopulmonary segment resection* is a "lung sparing" operation in which only the section of the lung lobe where the tumor is located is removed.[30]
- A *sleeve resection* is used if a tumor is in a main airway, or bronchus, with the tumor and surrounding tissue removed and both ends of the area closed with stitches.
- A *lobectomy*, commonly used for lung cancers, involves removal of the entire lobe of a lung containing cancerous tissue. A *pneumonectomy* involves removal of the entire lung. In many cases, this procedure has to be done via *thoracotomy* because of the size and location of the tumor.[31]

Pleural Effusion

Pleural effusion is the buildup of fluid in the pleural space—the area between the lungs and the chest wall. Ten to 50 percent of lung cancer patients develop pleural effusion. Cancer growing in the pleural space—common for people with non–small cell lung cancer (NSCLC)—causes a malignant pleural effusion (MPE), a condition in which fluid pushes against the lung, compressing and preventing it from fully expanding when breathing. Shortness of breath is the most common pleural effusion symptom, and the condition worsens as fluid accumulates.[32] This is exactly what happened to my patient Mary, whose case I discussed in the Preface.

More than 75 percent of people with a malignant pleural effusion have lung cancer. MPE is a metastatic disease hallmark, a clear indication that cancer has spread to other areas of the body, including the brain and bones. Malignant pleural effusion is treatable, but it shouldn't be taken lightly. It's a serious, usually life-threatening condition.

Thoracentesis is a procedure used to treat pleural effusion. During the procedure, a surgeon inserts a small tube (catheter) into the space around the lung, which allows for fluid drainage. Thoracentesis can usually be performed in a doctor's office or hospital room under local anesthesia by someone experienced using imaging to guide catheter placement. Thoracentesis provides immediate relief to patients, but it's just a quick fix. The fluid always reaccumulates to some degree. Some situations call for a thoracentesis, but, in my opinion, this procedure should only be performed once.

If the fluid reaccumulates, a more definitive procedure is needed. This involves leaving a pleural catheter within the chest cavity, which can be drained at home, allowing for optimal lung expansion and function. The catheter can be removed in the doctor's office once the fluid stops draining, allowing the lung to adhere to the chest wall and obliterating the space where the fluid is accumulating. Another procedure, *talc pleurodesis*, is used for the same purpose of getting the lung to adhere to the chest wall. I stopped performing talc pleurodesis many years ago because of the increased hospital stay and potential complications. The advantage of looking inside the chest with a camera (VATS) is that it determines whether the lung is touching the chest wall.

Mediastinal Tumors

Mediastinal tumors develop in the mediastinum, the area of the chest that separates the lungs and contains the heart, aorta, esophagus, and trachea. Although open surgery is occasionally necessary, VATS or robot-assisted techniques are an effective treatment for mediastinal tumors.

Side Effects of Lung Cancer Surgery

All surgery is trauma to the body, so you can expect any procedure, even one performed using minimally invasive techniques, to cause postoperative pain and put you at risk for complications. However, minimally invasive techniques reduce postoperative pain, enabling many patients to go home with just Tylenol and a heating pad. That's why it's in your best interests to seek out a minimally invasive surgeon.

Possible chest surgery complications include the following:

- Bleeding
- Infection

- Air leakage from the lung
- Pulmonary edema
- Complete or partial collapse of the lung or lobe of the lung (also called atelectasis)

Fortunately, in most cases, these complications can be managed with appropriate interventions. By decreasing pain with minimally invasive techniques, you can breathe deeper, get out of bed sooner, help inflate the lung, and recover quicker.

The Future Is Now: Lung Cancer Therapy Trends

Radiation Therapy Research

New techniques are in the works to enhance radiation therapy's effectiveness. I outline current trends in this section.

- **Radiosensitizers**
  Radiosensitizers are drugs that increase a cancer cell's sensitivity to the effects of radiation. Some radiosensitizers work by increasing cancer cells' oxygen levels because low levels of oxygen reduce radiation therapy's effectiveness. Some radiosensitizers disable tumor cells' DNA repair mechanisms, promoting cell death. Additional ways to increase cancer cell radiosensitivity are under investigation. Research suggests that radiotherapy, in conjunction with chemotherapy or as a stand-alone treatment, may offer the only possibility of cure for NSCLC.[33]
- **Radioprotectants**
  Limiting damage to healthy tissues in the treatment field is a great challenge facing radiotherapy. Radioprotectants are medicines that protect healthy tissues from radiation damage, thereby extending radiation's effectiveness on cancer cells and hopefully enhancing cancer control or elimination.[34]
- **Treatment Schedule Variations**
  Could it be that small, time-extended radiation doses are more effective than larger, short-term doses? That's the idea behind *fractionation*, the dividing or splitting of the total radiation dose into smaller doses. *Accelerated hyperfractionation*, arranging the treatment schedule so a patient receives three small, separate radiation doses per day, allows the total radiation dose to be delivered in a shorter time frame than would normally be called

for. Hyperfractionated and accelerated hyperfractionated treatment schedules are now used to treat NSCLC.[35-37]

• **Brachytherapy**
Unlike traditional radiotherapy, brachytherapy doesn't use external radiation, explaining why it's also referred to as internal radiation therapy. Brachytherapy is an advanced cancer treatment involving the placement of radioactive seeds in—or in close proximity—of the tumor itself, exposing it to a high radiation dose while reducing exposure to the surrounding healthy tissues. Brachytherapy is "short distance radiation therapy," meaning it's localized and precise. HDR brachytherapy, via catheters, provides a precise treatment that takes only a few minutes. This is not a standard treatment in lung cancer or mesothelioma, but ongoing studies indicate that it may reduce symptom severity and lengthen life.

• **Predicting Response to Therapy**
Scientists have the ability to test how well sample lung cancer tissue might respond to specific chemotherapy drugs. A large study involving more than 11,000 surgical patients with NSCLC found both adjuvant chemotherapy and adjuvant chemoradiotherapy increased the 5-year survival rate by 4 and 5 percent, respectively not huge numbers but still a noteworthy finding, especially for individuals facing a terminal diagnosis. There are questions about the overall testing accuracy and its effect on treatment outcomes. However, having accessible and reliable testing to predict the response of a specific cancer to certain drugs is a welcome development.[38]

• **Inhaled Chemotherapy**
Wouldn't it be great if cancer patients didn't have to spend hours in an uncomfortable chair with a needle stuck in their arm? Inhaled chemotherapy first surfaced 30 years ago, and recent animal studies have shown that it leads to a better rate of success against malignant lung tumors. Treatment of advanced lung cancer with conventional chemotherapy has been thwarted by toxicity and limited efficiency, with the chemotherapy causing systemic damage to healthy cells and organs and accumulating in the liver, kidney and spleen, rather than circulating to the target lungs. In contrast, a recent four-month animal study, published in the *Journal of Controlled Release*, demonstrated that 83 percent of lung tumors in mice treated with inhalation therapy disappeared, compared with 23 percent receiving intravenous injections.[39]

Inhalation therapy better destroyed resistant cancer cells, and more of the inhaled drugs reached the lungs than with traditional chemotherapy. Future studies are expected to show whether those advantages are demonstrated in human trials. The hope is that inhaled chemotherapy might one day be not only a more effective treatment, but also one that could be delivered to a patient at home.[40]

- **Targeted Therapy**
  Remember what I said earlier about chemotherapy drugs? Everything is fair game. They don't discriminate between tumor cells and healthy cells—they just act on all dividing cells. Targeted therapies are "molecularly targeted drugs," or more succinctly, "precision medicines" that precisely identify and attack cancer cells. Sparing normal cells is targeted therapy's goal.

THE MAGIC BULLET

One targeted therapy using a drug called crizotinib has been effective in patients when aimed at non–small cell cancer caused by a mutation in a particular gene, *ROS1*. The drug, marketed under the brand name Xalkori, showed a 72 percent response rate in patients with this mutation, according to a study published in the *New England Journal of Medicine*. The median response time was 19 months, which is considered a landmark in lung cancer treatment.[41]

Crizotinib has also been used in lung cancer patients with mutations of the *ALK* gene. In one study, people on crizotinib had more than double the survival rate compared with people on chemotherapy only. The impact of a drug like crizotinib proves that even in the presence of a rare mutation, the correct drug for the correct targets makes all the difference. Colon, stomach, brain, and gallbladder cancers also contain the *ROS1* mutation. Several clinical trials are under way to test targeted therapies on other mutation-triggered cancers.

A molecular-targeted therapy known as AZD9291 has made a difference in the treatment of advanced-stage lung cancer. The drug targets EGFR (epidermal growth factor receptor), a protein found on all cells, cancerous or not. In NSCLC cells, an EGFR mutation develops, leading to constant activation, uncontrolled cell division, and cancer growth. When individuals have lung cancer driven by EGFR, they at some point develop a tolerance to targeted treatment, which means it is no longer effective. This is often due to a T790M gene mutation, so treatment must return to the toxic therapies, such as chemotherapy and radiation. AZD9291 therapy in such cases most often results in a reduction in the size and growth of the NSCLC. Of the patients enrolled in one study who developed a resistance to previous medication and took AZD9291 once a day, 80 percent experienced tumor shrinkage or stability with manageable side effects.[42]

Table 5.1 contains examples of targeted therapy drugs for lung cancer that have been approved or are still in clinical trials.

- **Antiangiogenic Compounds**
  Like most living things, cancer cells need a steady blood supply to survive. Angiogenesis, the process of growing new blood vessels, is vital for cancer cells to go forth and multiply. Recent research has identified several antiangiogenic compounds that slow or inhibit the blood vessel growth process.[43] Two such compounds, endostatin and angiostatin, are the subject of clinical

Table 5.1.   Experimental Targeted Therapies for Lung Cancer

Generic Name	Trade Name	Target Activity
OSI-774, erlotinib	Tarceva	Anti-epidermal growth factor receptor (EGFR)
lonafarnib	Sarasar	Farnesyl transferase inhibitor
tipifarnib, R115777	Zarnestra	Farnesyl transferase inhibitor
imatinib	Gleevec	Tyrosine kinase inhibitor
ZD6474	Caprelsa	VEGF (vascular endothelial growth factor) receptor tyrosine kinase inhibitor
7-hydroxystaurosporine, UCN-01	—	G kinase inhibitor
suberoylanilide hydroxamic acid	Zolinza	Histone deacetylase (HDAC) inhibitor
bortezomib	Velcade	Proteasome inhibitor

Source: National Cancer Institute, The National Institutes of Health.

trials looking at the effectiveness of these and other antiangiogenic compounds in combination with standard lung cancer treatments.[44]

Thalidomide (Thalomid) received a lot of unwelcome notoriety in the 1950s because female cancer patients who took it to control side effects of nausea and vomiting later gave birth to babies with serious birth defects. However, it's the drug's antiangiogenic properties that arouse researchers' interests. Thalidomide has been used to successfully treat skin cancer and multiple myeloma, although there's still much debate surrounding its effectiveness as a treatment for lung cancer.[45]

A known angiogenesis inhibitor, Avastin, is already available to colon cancer patients. It's known to be useful for NSCLC patients but hasn't been used in large patient groups.[46] Also, researchers at Boston's Dana-Farber Cancer Institute found that Avastin, combined with standard NSCLC chemotherapy treatment, doesn't help lung cancer patients (65 years old and older) live longer.[47]

XL647 is another antiangiogenic drug undergoing clinical trials. XL647 binds and interacts with the vascular endothelial growth factor (VEGF) receptor involved in angiogenesis and the epidermal growth factor receptor, a receptor that is also a target for the cancer drugs Tarceva and Iressa.

Matrix metalloproteases (MMPs) are naturally occurring enzymes that help break down the structures between cells, making room for new, healthy tissue. New blood vessel development, tissue growth, and wound healing are important MMP-dependent processes, but cancer cells can use MMPs to migrate to distant tissue so new tumors can flourish.

MMP inhibitors (MMPIs) block the actions of MMPs. This treatment isn't without significant risks. Toxic side effects caused several clinical trials involving MMPIs to stop. BMS-275291 is currently the only MMPI in clinical trials. Still, the hunt continues for safe MMPIs that may slow or arrest lung cancer growth.

- **Antineoplastons**
These peptides, or small protein molecules, might return cancer cells to a normal cellular state. Scientist Stanislaw R. Burzynski first pinpointed and explained antineoplastons in 1976, but further study has yet to confirm his findings. The National Cancer Institute is now funding clinical studies of two among this

family of peptides, A10 and AS2-1, to determine what, if any, role they may play in cancer treatment.

Biological Therapies for Lung Cancer

You don't need to read this book to know that our immune system plays a major role in how well we respond to cancer. While terms like "biological therapy" or "immunotherapy" sound complicated, they're just umbrella terms for harnessing the immune system's cancer-fighting ability. Biological therapy, or "biological response modifier therapy" as it's sometimes called, is a newcomer to the cancer treatment community that uses the body's own immune system to fight disease. Vaccines or bacteria targeted to the body's immune system, aimed at triggering a more powerful immune system response to destroy cancer cells, are used in some therapies. Although these particular therapies don't target cancer cells directly, other biological therapies do. "Targeted therapies" interfere with specific molecules involved in tumor growth and spread. Because these therapies stimulate the body's response to infection and disease, they affect immune responses, as well as other critical bodily functions, and may even affect how we respond to cancer by preventing further disease spread.

- **Cytokines**
  Cytokines are naturally occurring "signaling" proteins produced by white blood cells that act as immune system messengers and mediators. Interferon, interleukin, and tumor necrosis factor are cytokines used to treat cancer patients. A fourth type, hematopoietic growth factor, counteracts chemotherapy's more adverse side effects. Cytokine therapy isn't without risk and carries significant side effects. Cytokine therapy is still not widely used.[48]
- **Monoclonal Antibodies**
  Antibodies are proteins running on borrowed time. They're manufactured by immune cells that attach to specific sites on cells, and each antibody type only affects a particular attachment site. Imagine a lock and key and you'll get a clear idea: Only one antibody (key) is effective with a specific site (lock). This quality makes them good vehicles for targeted cancer therapy because they attach to cancer cells but not normal cells. That is why they have been called "magic bullets" in the context

of monoclonal antibody therapy.[49] Trastuzumab (Herceptin), approved by the FDA to treat breast cancer, also binds to lung, prostate, and colon cancer cells. There are other monoclonal antibodies currently under investigation as possible lung cancer treatments, including the following:

- bevacizumab, rhuMab-VEGF (Avastin)
- cetuximab (Erbitux)
- LCG-Mab (lung cancer gene monoclonal antibodies)
- BEC2 (Mitumomab)
- TriGem
- anti-anb3 integrin (Medi-522)
- ABX-EGF

- **Immunotoxins**
  Immunotoxins are proteins composed of an antibody fragment linked to a toxin. They're used to treat cancer. Intratumoral anti-HuD immunotoxin therapy may be effective for SCLC and neuroblastoma.[50,51]
- **Immunoconjugates**
  Immunoconjugates, or antibody-drug conjugates, deliver chemotherapy only to cancer cells, while sparing healthy cells. SGN-15, which delivers the chemotherapy drug doxorubicin, is an immunoconjugate currently in clinical trial. According to an article recently published in the journal *Lung Cancer,* SGN-15, along with chemotherapy, may improve NSCLC patient outcomes.[52]
- **Cancer Vaccines**
  A vaccine is a dead or severely crippled agent such as a virus that produces immunity to a disease. Vaccines don't cure cancer, but they can reduce symptoms and even increase life expectancy in some patients.

Could Cuba's Lung Cancer Vaccine Help U.S. Patients?

Have you heard of CimaVax EGF? If not, perhaps you should get better acquainted. CimaVax EGF is the first Cuban-developed lung cancer vaccine, and it holds great promise. When President Obama loosened the reins in December 2016 on the United States' 55-year-long trade embargo against the island nation, he effectively paved the way for this miracle drug, which, after

25 years of research, became available free of charge to the Cuban citizens in 2011. In April 2014, the Cuban Center for Molecular Immunology signed an agreement with the Roswell Park Cancer Institute in Buffalo, New York, to import CimaVax EGF and begin clinical trials in the United States.[53]

Cuba, legendary for its high-quality and expensive cigars, has long lived under the specter of lung cancer, the country's fourth leading cause of death. A 2007 *Journal of Clinical Oncology* study of patients with advanced lung cancer confirmed CimaVax's safety and showed an increase in tumor-reducing antibody production in more than 50 percent of cases.[54] The vaccine was particularly effective for increasing survival in study participants younger than 60. To date, 5,000 patients worldwide have been treated with CimaVax, including 1,000 Cubans. Perhaps the best news of all: CimaVax is cheap and costs the Cuban government just $1.[55]

Chemoprevention

"Chemoprevention" is the use of medicines, vitamins, or other agents to prevent or delay the development of cancer. Unlike chemotherapy, chemoprevention medications are taken with the goal of avoiding cancer altogether, effectively eliminating the need for chemotherapy.

The treatments work differently, as well. Chemotherapy kills both healthy and malignant cells. Chemoprevention makes use of substances such as beta-carotene and vitamin E to prevent carcinogenesis. The *Journal of the National Cancer Institute* states that the "goal of chemoprevention is to inhibit the development of invasive cancer either by blocking the DNA damage that initiates carcinogenesis or by arresting or reversing the progression of premalignant cells in which such damage has already occurred."[56] There are three chemoprevention categories:

- *Primary prevention* is what it says. It's all about preventing malignancies in healthy people. These people may be at greater risk for lung cancer due to a history of smoking or specific genetic mutations.

Table 5.2. Substances with Lung Cancer Chemopreventive Potential

Nonsteroidal Antiinflammatory Drugs (NSAIDs)

Aspirin

Ibuprofen

Sulindac (Clinoril)

Celecoxib (Celebrex)

Rofecoxib (Vioxx)

Retinoids (Vitamin A Derivatives) and Carotenoids

9-cis-retinoic acid

Lutein

Zeaxanthin

13-cis-retinoic acid

  N-4-hydroxyphenyl retinamide (4-HPR) all-trans retinoic acid (ATRA)

Lycopene

Bexarotene

TAC-101

6-[3-(1-adamantyl)-4-hydroxyphenyl]-2-naphthalene carboxylic acid
(CD437) inhaled retinyl palmitate

Targeted Agents

Farnesyl transferase inhibitors ZD1839 (Iressa), tyrosine kinase inhibitor

Nutritional Supplements

Selenium

Vitamins C, D, and E

N-acetylcysteine (NAC) polyphenols (from green and black teas)

Curcumin (from the spice turmeric)

Allyl sulfur compounds (as in garlic)

Isothiocyanates myoinositol

Anethole dithiolethione (ADT, Sialor)

4-methyl-5-pyrazinyl-3H-1, 2-dithiolw-3-thione (oltipraz) terpenes
(found in cherries and lavender)

Limonene (found in citrus fruits, black pepper, and mangoes)

- *Secondary prevention* uses medications or vitamins to prevent the progression of cancer in patients with precancerous lesions.
- Preventing new cancer in patients cured of an initial cancer or individuals who have been treated for premalignant lesions is the focus of *tertiary prevention.*[57]

Radiofrequency Ablation

Radiofrequency ablation (RFA) is a nonsurgical, localized treatment that kills tumor cells while sparing healthy lung tissue. RFA is considered an alternative to systemic therapy for patients with small tumors because the treatment can be administered without adversely affecting the patient's overall health. During the procedure, a small needle is inserted through the skin into the tumor. Radiofrequency energy is transmitted from the needle tip, where it heats and kills the tumor tissues. The FDA has approved RFA for the treatment of tumors in soft tissues that include the lung.[58]

Cryoablation

While RFA uses heat to destroy tumors, cryoablation uses cold gas, delivered through the same kind of probe through the skin, to kill tumors. Although the procedure is well established, only recently have the probe needles been reduced enough in size to be used by interventional radiologists. Once inserted, the small needle injects what becomes an "ice ball," which expands to destroy the frozen tumor cells.[59]

Chemoembolization

When the tumor is not effectively treatable with RFA alone or with other treatments due to its location, chemoembolization becomes an option. Chemoembolization allows for a higher dose of chemotherapy to be used because the technique also keeps more of the cancer-killing drug from circulating to other, healthy cells where it may damage them. The chemotherapy, where a radiologist threads a very small catheter into an artery in the groin and to the blood vessel feeding the lung tumor, uses imaging to guide the catheter, and includes an embolizing agent. This agent controls the cancer-killing drug and keeps it in the tumor, while depriving it of its growth-inspiring blood supply by blocking arteries that would otherwise deliver blood to it.

Patients usually remain in the hospital for up to four days and experience lowered energy levels for up to 30 days. Although chemoembolization is palliative treatment, it has shown promise with some types of metastatic tumors.[60]

Gene Therapy

Gene therapy is used to increase cells' healthy genes. These may replace others that have been destroyed or damaged by a cancer, and, in the latter case, may bar expression of those damaged cells. Gene therapy was first tested in clinical trials 25 years ago. Recently, gene therapy has been used to treat Parkinson's disease, among many other conditions. Of great hope to thousands of lung cancer patients is a recent announcement that gene therapy may be an effective treatment for lung adenocarcinoma, which accounts for 40 percent of all lung cancers. To this point, lung adenocarcinoma has resisted targeted therapies. However, a research team at the Dana Farber Cancer Institute using two established drugs was able to stop the growth of this lethal lung cancer subtype in laboratory and animal studies. Human trials are expected in the near future.

Some adenocarcinomas carry mutations in the gene *KRAS*. Instead of targeting the *KRAS* gene itself, researchers set their sights on the *KRAS* genes' accomplices, or the genes that carry out the boss's instructions. Researchers were able to block something known as "cytokine signaling," which plays a role in cancer survival and the spread of the *KRAS* mutation. This new therapy basically eliminates lung adenocarcinoma's biggest survival strategy.

Major Advances in Lung Cancer Treatment

This time has been nothing but extraordinary. It's so fundamentally different from when I began my career more than 17 years ago, accelerating particularly over the past decade. Where we once had so few therapeutic options, we now have many more. We can now find tumors sooner. We can resect for cure using minimally invasive techniques. We have new drugs that target tumor cells. And we have more precise radiation therapy. Clearly, the goal is to find lung cancer in the earliest stages so we can cure it.

Across the last two decades, the treatment landscape has also been revolutionized by new drugs and classes of drugs, including taxanes and pemetrexed.[61] A decrease in the toxicity of therapies is a second major advance. Twenty years ago, every patient received the chemo-therapy drug, cisplatin. Our ability to control nausea and vomiting, probably the two biggest chemotherapy side effects, is much better today. Today, fewer and fewer patients experience nausea and emesis. Remember, you can always stop chemotherapy.

The use of targeted therapies is another big change on the horizon. How great would it be to choose treatments that were all but guaranteed to work for patients? Discovering the drivers that affect metabolism, and coming up with drugs that specifically target those changes and negate the cancer-causing and cancer-maintaining effects of these oncogenes, has been a paradigm-shifting development. Less toxicity factors in as well. The average Joe receiving targeted therapies finds them easier to take than traditional cytotoxic chemotherapies.

It's unwise to ever do away with effective treatments. Even today, virtually every lung cancer patient, including those receiving targeted therapies, receives cytotoxic intravenous chemotherapy. Fortunately, chemotherapy is no longer the only treatment of choice, and thousands of patients can—and do—live for long stretches without chemotherapy.

Even chemotherapy drugs like pemetrexed and bevacizumab are much easier to take—so much easier than cisplatin. In many ways, the best thing about pemetrexed is that it makes cisplatin a much easier drug to tolerate. By using these drugs, particularly the targeted drugs, and thus improving cure rates, we've moved the median. Still, we haven't changed cure rates to anywhere near the degree that we want for patients. That's the next frontier.

Future Promises: Better Cure Rates

Opportunities abound in the lung cancer treatment field. First to emerge from the fray are T-cell checkpoint inhibitors. These agents clearly induce important, durable, tolerable remissions. They need to be integrated quickly into the care of each and every patient. Unfortunately, we don't yet have a marker that can help us choose which patients are most likely to respond to those drugs. That's going to be the focus of research.[62] In the meantime, do what you can. Get a CT scan. Find out what's going on inside your chest and find someone who can explain it to you. Mention screening and mention minimally invasive surgery. Find it early and get rid of it.

The second opportunity has to do with targeted therapies. Today we can lengthen times to recurrence and also improve survival by giving targeted therapies only to those patients who have oncogenic drivers in their tumors.[63]

Where patients were once hospitalized just to receive treatment, many never have to be hospitalized at all. The lives of cancer patients are so much better today, and much less disrupted by therapy.

Pulling It All Together

Lung cancer is complex and there are no easy answers when it comes to making treatment decisions. There is no lung cancer treatment "gold standard." The practice of medicine is both a science and an art, and a guideline recommendation doesn't mean, under any circumstances, that the suggested treatment is your best option. Each person with lung cancer is different. The disease doesn't manifest the same in any two people. Because each person's system, circumstances, and needs vary, it is vital that lung cancer treatment is specifically designed for each patient. Ensure that your cancer care team knows your medical history, is aware of all the specifics of your case, and knows the best and most effective treatment options. When this is the case, the team will make the best recommendations. However, the ultimate power and authority ultimately rests with you.

CHAPTER 6

Complementary and Alternative Healing for Lung Cancer

Takeaways

- Complementary and alternative medicine (CAM) has been around for thousands of years, far longer than traditional allopathic (Western) medicine. Integrative medicine, which combines standard medicine and CAM, is a relatively new healing art, focusing not only on the disease but also the therapeutic relationship and the whole person.
- Almost 40 percent of U.S. adults use some type of CAM, usually to treat conditions for which Western medicine doesn't have easy answers, such as chronic pain, cancer, hepatitis C, and a number of other intractable conditions. Medicinal herbs, dietary supplements, mind–body practices like yoga and meditation, and massage are the most frequently used CAM therapies.
- CAM techniques such as acupuncture and massage are thought to be helpful for relieving pain and nausea, two common side effects of lung cancer treatment.
- Fear of judgment causes many patients to hide their interesting usage of CAM. Therefore, it's the responsibility of physicians to ask their patients about CAM in a nonjudgmental fashion. Physicians must be able to determine whether seemingly "harmless" CAM approaches—such as certain therapies or nutritional supplements may actually pose harm because of how they might interact with cancer treatment drugs. Physicians can guide patients to qualified, respected CAM providers, and also track progress or spot any problems early. That tracking also benefits education and research that can help future patients.

Introduction

What does it mean to be healthy? That's a question I'm often asked. I've practiced medicine for more than 17 years, but to this day, I still fumble for an answer. I'd like to say that "healthy" is the absence of disease, infirmity, or disability, but that's not really true. There are physically healthy people, free of any identifiable illness, that barely function. I remember treating a patient with a collapsed lung. Today, five years after surgery, she's illness-free but chronically depressed. On the other end of the spectrum, I have a Stage III lung cancer patient who's productive at work and enjoys a close, loving relationship with his wife and three children. Who's healthier? When it comes to our health, quality, not quantity, matters most.

Indeed, good health implies more than the "absence of disease." The word "health" (heal) refers to the state of "being whole," which implies being or becoming a whole person—physically, mentally, and spiritually. I could argue that death is natural and part of our true self since it's an inevitable part of the human condition.

Sure, I can remove a lung mass, preach the prevention gospel, and lecture about the dangers of smoking. But is this enough? Because we can do something doesn't always mean we should do something. Gary Ratson, M.D., author of *The Meaning of Health*, used to ask his medical school instructors and advisors if the patients they treated were healthier after treatment. Dr. Ratson's question, which must have annoyed many of his teachers, raise an interesting point about our lowered expectations for optimal health.[1]

The medical establishment's consideration of the emotional, social and spiritual aspects of a patient's well-being is relatively new phenomenon. Dr. William Osler, one of the founding fathers of Johns Hopkins Hospital, said it best, "It's more important to know what sort of person has the disease than what sort of disease has the person."

Until now, we've spoken extensively about the physical manifestations of lung cancer and lung cancer treatment. This chapter considers a much broader definition of "health."

Healing Systems

Western Medicine

Western medicine is relatively new branch of healing. Hippocrates (460–370 BC), universally recognized as the father of Western medicine, proposed a new model that relied on natural, rather than supernatural, explanations of illness. The Hippocratic treatise *On the Sacred Disease*, which was probably authored not only by Hippocrates, but several like-minded practitioners, opens with the following: "[epilepsy] appears to me to be nowise more divine nor more sacred than other diseases, but has a natural cause from which it originates like other affections."[2] Western medicine remains evidence based, its methodology fundamentally analytical and reductive. Using algorithms of signs and symptoms, allopathic medical doctors sort patients into disease categories. Generally, although not always, treatments come into play after they have been scientifically tested—a process that takes years and often fails—for efficacy and safety, meaning they were shown to be effective for a specific disease or condition in published peer-reviewed scientific literature.

At the Other End of the Spectrum

Complementary and alternative medicine (CAM) is a rubric referring to many healing systems that fall outside the realm of traditional allopathic medicine. Unlike allopathic medicine, CAM therapies are rarely used as a standalone treatment in the United States. More often, they complement, or are used in conjunction with, allopathic medicine. Dr. Mehmet Oz, for an example, was one of the first clinicians to introduce meditation into the operating room, and Jon Kabat-Zinn, an MIT-trained molecular biologist, is credited with being the first Western-trained scientist to integrate yoga, meditation, and other mindfulness practices with traditional allopathic medical interventions. Together, allopathic and conventional medicine is referred to as *integrated* medicine. Alternative therapy, as the names suggests, sometimes eschews conventional treatment altogether.[3] Some holistic practitoners do accept or use the traditional medical model when necessary. Many people use alternative methods only after conventional treatments fail when they're given a diagnosis for which no medically recognized treatment exists. Better yet, more and more people are using CAM as a prophylactic measure, hoping never to become unhealthy. However, with all the recent advances in conventional allopathic medicine, especially in the field of cancer treatment, patients' doctors must make sure that patients know the possible dangers of using CAM in lieu of Western therapy.

While researching the CAM therapies most used by lung cancer patients, I have made sure to see if there is credible scientific evidence supporting a particular treatment or product. At the present time, and for a number of reasons, including major-league financial hurdles, the majority of CAM therapies have not been studied in a clinical setting, meaning there'll be no scientific study proving their effectiveness. Anecdote and tradition are the basis for the effectiveness, or ineffectiveness, of most CAM therapies. And because we still don't understand the underlying mechanisms of a number of allopathic medical treatments, doctors routinely fall back on intuition in making treatment recommendations.[4]

I can't, as a reputable physician, provide an endorsement here on the effectiveness of CAM treatments. Patients regularly solicit my opinions on the effectiveness of alternative cancer treatments, many of which I'd never even heard of until I started writing this book. Because my discussion is limited to lung cancer, I can't support CAM in lieu of traditional medicine. They show up for office consults lugging bags of "cancer fighting" supplements and vitamins, convinced that somewhere deep inside their magic bag there lies that yet-to-discovered cancer cure. My personal opinions don't matter. My job is to present information—good, bad, and neutral. The inclusion of a particular therapy or treatment shouldn't be taken as a ringing endorsement. Similarly, exclusion of a particular CAM treatment doesn't mean I'm opposed to it or I think it doesn't work. On the contrary, I've seen some, albeit limited, scientific evidence that a handful of CAM therapies may work better, or at least as well as, some conventional modalities.

Before adding a new therapy to your treatment plan, please discuss your intentions with your lung cancer care team. Any therapy, whether CAM or standard Western treatment, can interfere with the positive effects of other treatments. Foods, vitamins, supplements, herbs, and homeopathic drugs can interact with conventional treatments to not only increase effectiveness but also to increase negative side effects. Some combinations can be very harmful and even deadly.[5] Because many CAM treatments aren't covered by health insurance, use caution before trying these costly and often unproven therapies.

What should you look for in a CAM practitioner or therapy? The following is my checklist of the top 10 things to weigh when considering CAM. This same list could easily apply to conventional allopathic medicine as well.

1. What's the CAM provider's background? There's some major real estate separating allopathic doctors from acupuncturists, especially when it comes to lung cancer.

2. How much experience does the provider bring to the table?
3. Is he or she certified or licensed to practice in his field? Keep in mind, however, that this doesn't always equate to treatment effectiveness or ensure that the practitioner is a good therapist.
4. What's the out-of-pocket cost, since many CAM treatments aren't covered by insurance?
5. If insurance is in play, does it cover all, or even part of the cost?
6. Will the treatment you're considering move you closer to your desired outcome?
7. What are the goals of the therapy you're considering?
8. What are the risks and side effects associated with this therapy? (If the treatment is truly effective, there will be some.)
9. Has the treatment been evaluated in clinical trials or undergone rigorous scientific testing? This doesn't mean, however, that it will or won't work but only that it's been subjected to scientific scrutiny. Have the findings been published in peer-reviewed journals or presented at a scientific conference?
10. How will the treatment affect other therapies you're receiving? Remember, if your treatment is powerful enough to help or heal, the converse must also be true: they are powerful enough to harm as well.

Popular Complementary and Alternative Therapies for Lung Cancer

Ayurveda

The term "Ayurveda" is a merger of the Sanskrit words *ayur* (meaning "life") and *veda* (meaning "knowledge") and dates back thousands of years, making it one of the world's oldest healing systems. The health of the digestive system and digestive functions are central of Ayurveda. Ayurvedic medicine aims to maximize mental and emotional health by facilitating good diet, exercise, herb use, detoxifying or "cleansing" the body, and other approaches

Ayurvedic principles state that each person is imbued with three vital energies, or *doshas*, that give us each a unique constitution—*vata*, *pitta*, and *kapha*. A balance of the three *doshas* is needed for optimal health. Ayurvedic medicine isn't widely studied in the West, and the United States doesn't license ayurvedic practitioners. Predictably, there's scant scientific literature supporting the use of Ayurveda.

Chiropractic

I've never had lung cancer, but I did try chiropractic to great effect. I tried chiropractic to great effect after Cincinnati Reds legend and Hall of Fame catcher Johnny Bench convinced me that a few little adjustments could relieve pressure on my chronically inflamed sciatic nerve. The treatment worked, much to my surprise and delight. This is not an endorsement of chiropractic for lung cancer treatment, I'm just honoring its possible effectiveness for non-life-threatening conditions.

Chiropractic medicine is all about the relationship between body structure—specifically the spine—and functioning. Chiropractic treatment is based on the idea that the nervous system controls all bodily functions—it does—and spinal misalignments disrupt these functions. Chiropractic doctors use a number of treatment modalities, including electrical stimulation, and ice, but the primary intervention involves manipulating, or adjusting the spine or other parts of the body to alleviate pain, improve function, and support the body's innate healing abilities.[6] Chiropractic, in conjunction with conventional medicine, may be beneficial for alleviating some lung cancer-related symptoms, but shoud never be used in lieu of.

Homeopathy

Dr. Samuel Hahnemann, a German doctor and pharmacist, developed homeopathic medicine almost 200 years ago. Like other alternative remedies, homeopathy claims to treat the whole person rather than just a symptom(s). Homeopathy is based on the principle that "like treats (or cures) like," something known as the principle of similar, and the "law of minimum dose," which, just as the name implies, holds that the lower the dose, the more effective the medication. Homeopathic remedies, which consist of small doses of harmful stuff, supposedly stimulate the body's natural healing systems. The Food and Drug Administration (FDA) regulates homeopathic remedies, and they're manufactured by established pharmaceutical companies under strict guidelines.[7]

Understand that, as with Ayurveda, in the United States homeopathic practitioners are not licensed or regulated, so there is no federal credentialing or quality control. State laws do not exist for controlling it either, with the exception of one state, Arizona. Other states allow homeopathy within the scope of practice for specific health professions such as acupuncture.[8]

But does homeopathy even work? Some experts claim it's ineffective and even dangerous if used as a substitute for proven, conventional remedies. An analysis of 225 studies and 1,800 research papers by Australian researchers really took the wind out of the alternative medical community's collective sail, concluding that there are "no health conditions for which there is reliable evidence that homeopathy is effective."

Naturopathy

Naturopathy combines natural, nontoxic therapies (not all natural therapies are nontoxic, I might add) with more conventional therapies and can rightfully lay claim to the "integrative medicine" moniker. Naturopathy is all about tapping the source, as practitioners believe that the body has an inborn self-healing ability. Naturopathic medicine looks for the underlying cause of a particular illness instead of focusing solely on treatment/palliation of symptoms. Naturopathic doctors receive rigorous training in many disciplines, allowing them to try and number of therapeutic approaches to support self-healing. Diet, exercise, nutrition, massage, acupuncture, homeopathic remedies, herbal medicines, and nutritional supplements all fall under the naturopathy rubric. Whole-patient wellness, disease prevention, and self-care are the focus of this discipline.

Traditional Chinese Medicine

Traditional Chinese medicine (TCM) is a 3,000-year-old healing system that grounds its understanding of health and healing on natural law. According to TCM principles, the human body always is working to reconcile, or strike a balance between, opposing forces such as hot and cold, damp and dry, and masculine and feminine. Thus, optimal health is achieved when there is a balance between the body's opposing forces, known also as yin and yang. Disease, on the other hand, results from imbalances. Qi (pronounced "chee") is a vital energy that travels along meridians, the body's internal pathways. Imbalances block the flow of qi, which practitioners correct by using a number of modalities.

Complementary Healing and Cancer

In Western medicine, cancer is the primary disease-causing problem. Alternative medical practitioners have a slightly different view, not surprisingly. Cancer arises, say many, from underlying problems that have provided fertile soil for cancer to flourish. Western medical treatment focuses on killing cancer cells; alternative therapies rid the body of cancer by restoring and supporting overall health.

Attention paid to the "whole person" is another distinguishing feature of the CAM approach. In Western medicine, the focus is always on the physical aspects of health and disease. Allopathic medical practitioners integrate nonphysical practices into their treatment paradigms, but the primary focus still is physical health and disease management. CAM disciplines take a broader approach, believing that a key to well-being can be found by looking at the complex interactions among mind, body, and spirit, meaning that one can only be physically well if there's a balance between this holy trinity.

Allopathic (Western) medicine, CAM, or an integrated approach—it's really your choice. I just want readers to be aware of all options for treatment. Of course, there are caring alternative medicine practitioners dedicated to helping people heal and be as well as possible, but there are a few whose motives may not be as altruistic or well educated. CAM therapies aren't often subject to the kinds of clinical trials demanded of Western medicine. Consumers may be taking a risk if they rely on unscientific, anecdotal assurances and unsupported theories in lieu of a conventional lung cancer treatment program, particularly with late-stage disease. Be sure to consult your physician first if you are considering alternative medicine.

Common Concepts

CAM therapies share many concepts and jargon. Following are two of the most common.

Mind–Body Interactions　There's little doubt that mind–body interactions affect health and disease. Across the board, CAM disciplines aggressively promote this idea. A number of complementary and alternative therapies for lung cancer (e.g., meditation, yoga, and biofeedback) focus equally on physical health and psychological well-being.

Optimizing Immune Function　The immune system is a critical player in our response to cancers. T lymphocytes (T cells)—specialized white cells—natural killer cells, and macrophages work together, seeking out and destroying cancer cells. CAM cancer treatments are designed to maximize and support immune system function. Optimizing the body's natural ability to heal itself from cancer is the treatment goal.

Optimizing Immune Function: Separating Science Fiction from Science Fact

How often have you heard someone talking about how a certain food or supplement can boost your immune system? It's certainly a question patients raise with me. I'm not sure how to respond, honestly, and wish the answer were as simple as, "Add this food or supplement to your diet."

The human immune system is remarkably complex, a still not fully understood network of organs, tissues, biomolecules, and cells that work in tandem to ward off a constant daily onslaught of pathogens. "Experts" can tell you to eat this super food (there's no such thing) or pop this supplement to ward off disease, but in a great majority of cases, these interventions do nothing except empty your wallet.

For sure, there are a number of chronic conditions, such as diabetes, that reduce our body's ability to ward off illnesses that have an impact on immune system response. There also are a number of people who are born with an impaired immune response, and a number of medical treatments—most famously chemotherapy—that weaken or even destroy the immune system. However, garden-variety infections don't weaken the immune system. Indeed, the "sick feeling" patients complain of during a cold or flu is usually part of the normal immune response.

Patients should heed the usual guidance to eat right, exercise, get adequate rest, and manage stress, there really isn't an effective way make the immune system better. And there are even reasons why an overactive or too powerful immune system is a bad thing. A "cytokine storm" is a potentially lethal immune reaction that occurs when too many immune cells are activated in a single place, such as an infection site.[9] An overactive immune system can also attack the host body's cells, leading to nasty autoimmune diseases such as rheumatoid arthritis.

To be honest, I still haven't seen a whole lot of evidence that a normally functioning immune system can be successfully boosted.

And here's a final thing worth knowing about the human immune system: It's pretty resilient. If our immune systems were as awful as some claim, few of us would make it make it past infancy. So the next time someone suggests you "boost your immune system," you might respond by asking, "which part?"

Detox The practice of "detox" or detoxification is a mainstay of many complementary and alternative healing paradigms. The premise is that a host of environmental toxins may be contributing to the cancerous process. Detoxification treatments, of which there are dozens, allegedly remove toxins from the body, restoring normal bodily function, and eliminating the negative effects of repeated exposures.

Can You Really Detox Your Body?

It's an interesting concept. I mean, the idea that you can wash away effects of your unhealthy habits and repeated environmental exposure to noxious chemicals with a weeklong juice fast or by strategically placing a long red tube up your rectum. But take heed. Before you plunk down a couple hundred bucks on the latest newfangled juicer promoted by someone who really has no business talking to you about anything remotely medical, consider this fact: The $5 billion cleanse industry is almost certainly a scam designed to part you from your hard-earned money.

In medicine, there is, of course, such a thing as detox, but it's accomplished by the skin, liver, kidneys, colon and lungs, or it's reserved for treating drug addicts. The other, and incredibly lucrative, detox business may be a mythological landscape consisting of pseudoscientific nonsense that passes as real medical advice and is nearly always promoted by charlatans who insist their treatment can rid your body of the toxins—ingested, inhaled, or absorbed poisonous substances—it accumulates. Listen up, folks, your body has its own built-in detox system, consisting of the aforementioned lungs, kidneys, colon, liver, and skin, which work in tandem 24/7 to rid your body of anything it doesn't need or anything that might cause it harm. If the opposite were true, you'd be as dead as Julius Caesar. Perhaps I'm missing something, but to my knowledge, there isn't a way—that means there's no tea, supplement, pill, miracle diet, or special massage—to make your body's natural detox system work any better than it already does. And some popular detox staples can actually do more harm than good. Even the much-heralded, nutrient-rich broccoli, which, like all plants from the *Brassica* genus, contains cyanide, equips the liver to better deal with the daily poison onslaught, but it can be harmful in large amounts.

If you really want to detox, stop smoking (if you haven't already), lay off the donuts, quit drinking alcohol, get some exercise, and practice stress management. This is enough for most people, even lung cancer patients. This disease is hard enough. Why punish yourself just trying to be healthy?

Nutrition We all know the saying "You are what you eat." But a more accurate way to put it, in the view of complementary and alternative therapies, is "Your health is what you eat." CAM and alternative medicine therapies often focus on patients getting the best nutrition in order to have top normal function and to heal from disease and disorders, including cancer. Certainly, a diet rich in cheese puffs, potato chips, and cupcakes isn't going to meet your nutritional needs, whether you have cancer or not. But nutrition's value both as a cancer fighter and preventer remains an open question. Linda McCartney, the first wife of superstar Paul McCartney and a longtime vegetarian and healthy eating advocate, died of breast cancer. This isn't to imply that a healthy diet, whatever that may be since there's really no consensus as to what constitutes a healthy diet, isn't a good idea for lung cancer patients, or people in general. Rather, there are many factors that contribute to the development and spread of cancer, and we shouldn't rely solely on the promise of miracle foods to cure what ails us.

Stress Reduction and Emotional, Mental, and Spiritual Health

There's an ample body of evidence that nonphysical factors influence health and disease. In this section, I've listed a number of healing techniques that emphasize stress reduction or emotional and mental well-being. There are other techniques available, but I have only included those most often used by cancer patients.

Art Therapies

Some cancer patients turn to art therapy to find stress relief, relax, and gain a sense of well-being. These therapies may include making music

or art, dance and other creative movement, and dramatic performance. Advocates say it is part of a mind–body approach, so what
threatens the health of one can sooner or later weaken the other, and
what relaxes, strengthens, or otherwise empowers one can do the
same for the other.

Supporters say activities such as these, often directed by psycholo-
gists or mental health counselors, foster human development and
psychological health. In the process of creativity, clients can find self-
esteem, resolve emotional problems, develop self-awareness, reduce
anxiety, and get perspective that helps them increase self-esteem, as
well as meet others and discover new supports and abilities by developing new social skills. Feelings and psychological conflicts, for example, may be vented and sorted out on canvas, in music, or on the
dance floor. Art therapy is practiced at hospitals, psychiatric and rehabilitation facilities, wellness centers, forensic institutions, schools,
crisis centers, and senior centers.[10]

The American Dance Therapy Association defines dance/movement
therapy as, "the psychotherapeutic use of movement as a process which
furthers the emotional, cognitive and physical integration of the individual."[11] I have a patient who died recently after a long struggle with
Stage IV non–small cell lung cancer. She outlived her oncologist's prognosis and was still going strong four years after her initial diagnosis.
She credited her ability to defy the odds to her lifelong passion for
ballet, in which she continued to perform until she entered hospice
care. True, this is an anecdotal account, but I do believe that having
something in her life that she cared deeply about helped my patient
defy the odds and live well beyond what many of us expected.

Music therapy has generated a number of headlines recently for its
ability to positively affect executive functioning in children with
learning and emotional/psychological problems. It may play an
equally important role in physical rehabilitation, movement facilita-
tion, and improved motivation—critical for cancer patients—and
may even serve as an emotional outlet for patients and their families.
A 2010 study found that 42 percent of hospitalized patients who
listened to familiar music for just 30 minutes a day saw a 50 percent
improvement in their pain threshold. Many cancer patients find music therapy helpful as part of their overall treatment plan.[12]

Drama therapy, the "systematic and intentional use of drama/
theater processes, products, and associations to achieve the therapeutic goals of symptom relief, emotional and physical integration and
personal growth," can help patients tell their stories, solve problems,

and release their feelings. Lung cancer patients face many challenges that drama therapy may help them work through. A report out of London's King's College Hospital found that the anxiety levels of brain cancer patients either stayed the same or decreased after participation in a six-week drama program and that all participants expressed interest in attending support groups for their condition after finishing the program.[13]

A meta-analysis of 27 studies involving almost 1,600 people found that study participants who got involved in creative arts therapy reported less pain, depression, and anxiety than other cancer patients who did not get involved. Overall, they said their quality of life improved while they were using creative arts therapy.[14] The benefits of creative arts therapy were similar to those reported by cancer patients who participated in integrative cancer services including acupuncture and yoga.

Biofeedback

Biofeedback is a technique people use to control their body functions and improve their health. Most body functions such as heartbeat take place, for the most part, outside of conscious awareness. During biofeedback, an EEG (electroencephalography) machine records the brain's electrical activity, which appears as continuous waves on a piece of paper, to help a patient gain dominion over specific body functions, like breathing and heart rate. I've treated a number of lung cancer patients who successfully used biofeedback to control anxiety, stress, breathing problems, and pain. The therapy is not without its detractors, and a number of studies have found that biofeedback isn't any more effective than conventional therapies for a number of common ailments.[15, 16]

Hypnosis

There's a lot of myth surrounding the practice of hypnosis. If you think about it, hypnosis may just be part of our natural state. Have you ever been oblivious to the world around you? If so, isn't that really the equivalent of a hypnotic trance? How about driving and suddenly realizing you're 20 miles closer to your destination? A hypnotized person is awake, but not actively engaged in the normal habits. We pass through a similar state right before we wake up or fall asleep.

Can hypnotherapy help the cancer patient? There's evidence suggesting that hypnotherapy can be helpful when used alongside conventional medical treatments. In particular, hypnotherapy may be a useful adjunct for reducing cancer-related pain, anxiety, insomnia, nausea, and vomiting. Hypnosis isn't recommended for patients with co-occurring mental illness such as schizophrenia or dementia.[17]

Massage

Massage therapy treats the body's soft tissues, primarily muscle and connective tissues using different techniques, which, if used correctly, can positively affect the circulatory, musculoskeletal, nervous, and respiratory systems. Of interest to cancer patients are massage's positive effects—disability prevention, stress and pain relief. Hydrotherapy, stretching and strengthening exercises, breathing instruction, and postural assessment and alignment are other tools massage therapists use as part of their treatment protocols.

How effective is massage for relieving common cancer symptom and treatment side effects? A review of 14 trials suggested that massage can help reduce a number of disease-related symptoms including "pain, nausea, anxiety, depression, anger, stress and fatigue." But the reviewers also cited the "poor quality" of certain trials and said it wasn't possible to know for certain and to what degree massage helped with cancer symptoms.[18]

There are many forms of massage therapy. Following are some common massage forms:

Acupressure Acupressure, or *tui na*, is acupuncture, just without the needles. Rooted in traditional Chinese medicine that has been practiced for thousands of years, acupressure aims to relieve pain and stiffness when the a practitioner applies pressure to certain points of the body with his or her fingers, palms, or elbows. Chinese theory holds that the pressure promotes ideal flow of the life force known as qi, described earlier in the section on TCM. A common Western view is that any positive results stem from reduced muscle tension, better blood flow, and or acupressure's stimulation of the release of the body's natural painkillers, called endorphins.

Craniosacral Therapy Craniosacral therapy, or cranial osteopathy, is the brainchild of Dr. William Sutherland, and was later refined by the osteopathic physician and professor of biomechanics, John E.

Upledger. Sutherland was the first person to notice the pliability of the skull's synarthrodial joints (also known as cranial sutures). Practitioners apply light hand pressure to a person's skull, spine, and pelvis, which is thought to regulate the flow of cerebrospinal fluid. Cranial osteopathy is controversial because there's no real evidence to support its core assertion that the central nervous system emits "subtle, rhythmic pulsations" that can be detected and modified by a skilled practitioner—in this case, an osteopath. According to the American Cancer Society website, craniosacral therapy isn't a proven cancer treatment, but it may relieve stress and tension.

Deep-Tissue Massage   For chronic aches and pains, some cancer patients seek deep-tissue massage. In this technique, a practitioner uses his or her fingers, thumbs, or elbows to massage an area with slow, deep strokes, working into the muscle and connective tissue.

Lymph Drainage Massage   After chest surgery, some doctor may recommend lymph node drainage, which involves light, rhythmic strokes on the affected lymph nodes. This massage technique may improve poor lymph flow and reduce swelling following inflammation, edema, and peripheral neuropathy, all common lung cancer surgery side effects.[19]

Neuromuscular Massage   Neuromuscular massage, in which a practitioner's hands work over specific muscles, is thought to stimulate circulation and release tension, pressure, and nerve pain.[20] One form of this massage is known as "trigger point" therapy, in which finger pressure is applied to a tight area within muscle tissue that is believed to be causing pain in another part of the body.[21]

Reflexology   This form of massage is based on a system theorizing that points on the hands, feet, and ears correspond to other organs and systems throughout the body. The practitioner applies pressure to select points to promote health and healing in the corresponding body part. When appropriately administered, reflexology can reduce pain, anxiety, depression, and increase relaxation. Participants report that the treatment is generally relaxing and reduces stress. Reflexology practitioners include chiropractors, physical therapists, and massage therapists.

Rolfing   Rolfing is a form of deep tissue massage developed by biochemist Ida P. Rolf to reset alignment in the body, thereby restoring better movement and posture, reducing stress, and increasing well-being. Common areas of focus are the upper back, neck, and shoulders. Studies have shown that it may be beneficial for a number of neurological impairments.

Shiatsu   Like acupressure, shiatsu is based on the traditional Chinese medicine view that illness is believed to result from imbalanced life energy, or qi. Developed in Japan, shiatsu uses finger-pressure massage. The practitioner applies pressure with his or her fingers and palms, aiming to improve the flow of qi in the client's body. Shiatsu works by relaxing the sympathetic nervous system, improving circulation, relieving stiff muscles, injury recovery, aches and pains, and reducing stress. A 2008 European study noted that people receiving shiatsu reported overall positive changes in symptom severity and health-related behavior, suggesting a role for shiatsu in maintaining and enhancing health.[21] However, a 2011 review found little evidence supporting shiatsu's purported health benefits."[22]

Swedish Massage   The most popular form of massage in the United States, Swedish massage involves soft strokes and kneading, as well as light tapping strokes on the muscles. It includes soft movement of joints, muscles, and connective tissue. Among the benefits reported are pain relief, decreased anxiety, increased relaxation, and a greater sense of well-being. Studies are under way on the correlation between Swedish massage and reduction of fatigue in cancer patients, as well as reduction of anxiety and depression in patients with other chronic diseases.

Thai Massage   First developed in India more than 2,500 years ago by a man believed to be Gautama Buddha's personal physician, Thai massage is a variation on classical massage in which a therapist uses their hands, feet, and legs to move a client's body into a sequence of yoga-like poses; it also integrates techniques of acupressure. There is no scientific evidence that Thai massage has any therapeutic value for lung cancer patients. However, people feel better and report that Thai massage may relieve some cancer symptoms or help with treatment side effects.

Meditation

The human mind is a ceaseless source of activity, constantly fluctuating between thoughts, often negative and harmful. We do not summon those dark ones; they stream in of their own power—or so it seems. But people who have been trained in mediation learn to control what thoughts enter their minds, that is, how to slow or halt the "dark noise" and find a calm, peaceful state. Many cancer patients report that meditation helps rid them of unpleasant or destructive thoughts.

Visualization is a meditation hybrid in which a practitioner focuses on a specific image. A cancer patient, for an example, may visualize something he or she would like to see occur. Some patients may visualize themselves cancer free or picture their body's cancer cells dying. Others might visualize a happy place, time, or activity. *Guided Imagery* focuses on a particular object, except that someone—other than you—directs the visualization process, talking you through the experience. People often begin with guided imagery to learn the techniques and eventually practice self-directed visualization.

These are just two examples of the many meditation techniques available. According to the Meditation Society of America, there are 108 recognized meditation techniques, all variations on the same theme in that they mobilize unconscious and preconscious processes to quiet and focus the mind and improve well-being. Personality and temperament determine the technique. Don't assume meditation is easy, however. It's a discipline that requires time, practice, and commitment. Practitioners report that it inspires a mental clarity and peace that cancer patients may find very beneficial.

Mind–Body Exercise

Exercise has many benefits, all of which you're probably either familiar with or have even experienced directly.* Improved mood, stress relief, increased strength, stamina, and flexibility—it's not even necessary to list all the possible benefits. However, some exercise forms are more useful than others at achieving that all-elusive goal of mind–body union. Yoga is an ancient Indian practice dating back thousands of years. *Yoga* is one part, or limb, of an overall spiritual practice of mind–body control. There are many forms of yoga; some are very gentle, while others are extremely rigorous. Along with improving strength and flexibility, yoga practitioners say—and limited studies even suggest—that regular yoga practice improves a number

---

Please discuss any exercise program with your doctor or health care provider to be sure it's safe for you. Most of the exercises presented in this chapter are best learned from a qualified teacher.

of important bodily functions, while fostering emotional stability and clear thinking. The great thing about yoga is that anyone can practice it, regardless of his or her current weight or flexibility, and with minimal equipment and limited space.

Qi gong (pronounced chee gung) originated in China, and it incorporates visualization as well as slow movements, controlled breathing, and body positions. All are intended to help promote better flow of the blood and the life force (qi) throughout the body and brain. Positive effects sought include increased energy, stronger bodily functions, and a "cleansing" of body and mind. The breathing techniques of Qi gong are believed by practitioners to facilitate energy flow, open up meridians to all vital structures, and thus fuel healing. A related martial art, *tai chi*, uses similar, slow, gentle movements to improve health and build muscle tone. Like qi gong, tai chi increases qi or energy in the internal organs, releasing stress while improving balance and coordination. A study in the *Annals of Behavioral Medicine* found that both tai chi and qi gong improved cancer-related fatigue in breast cancer survivors but had no effect on mood and sleep disturbances.[23]

Support Groups

I love support groups. They're a life-giving resource for thousands of cancer patients. They help in a number of ways, but I especially like the fact that they provide an outlet for patients and their loved ones to express their emotions and help lessen the feelings of being alone with the experience of cancer. Most importantly, they foster a sense of hope, which is really what this book is all about.

Together or separately, support groups can help greatly reduce psychological distress and, simply put, make you feel better, more at ease, and stronger. They are especially vital for people with otherwise limited or absent supports. There are probably dozens of local and online support groups near you. Check with your local hospital, caregiver, or cancer association branch and see the resource section at the back of this book.

Nutritional Supplements

Simply, nutritional supplements—that is, vitamins, minerals, and other products—provide additional nutrients beyond those obtained through your diet. Cancer patients are a prime demographic for supplements manufacturers, and hundreds of products are marketed directly to them. In this climate, finding the right product can be challenging. *The Physicians' Desk Reference for Nonprescription Drugs and Dietary Supplements* (www.pdr.net) has a boatload of information about nutritional supplements.

In the next few pages, I review a handful of products that patients routinely ask me about. As a traditional allopathic medical doctor, I'm really on the fence about nutritional supplements. And I'm loath to recommend anything that hasn't been subjected to rigorous scientific scrutiny, which few products are for reasons that aren't important to expound upon in this type of book. Also, I don't advise my patients to research products they're considering since the Internet is a veritable factory of misinformation. My only advice is that you discuss any products you're considering with your physician or other health care provider, such as a dietician or nutritionist. I will offer one caveat, however. Supplements are weak drugs; this means that they, like all drugs, can and often do interact with other drugs and products, potentially interfering with treatments you're receiving and making them dangerous in the right combination. If you believe the manufacturer claims that these products are powerful enough to heal, then the converse should apply as well: they are also powerful enough to do harm.

Patients frequently change their nutritional intake after a cancer diagnosis. Some opt for a strictly organic diet or eschew animal protein, believing such products may be contributing to their illness. What's the right answer? Again, it depends who's doing the talking. One study found that middle-aged people on high-protein diets are more likely to die of cancer than those who eat less protein.[24] On the other hand, for people age 65 and over, moderate protein intake might entail certain benefits, such as offering protection against frailty. Whatever you decide, confer with a doctor or nutritionist and/ or dietician to be sure you are getting the calories and basic nutrients you need.

Let's get one more thing out of the way: The human body makes many of the nutrients it needs to carry out its functions. Some life-sustaining nutrients can't be made quickly enough—or at all, however. These "essential nutrients" can only be found in outside sources, including food and supplements. Cancer patient or not, human beings need six separate groups of essential nutrients, each vital for growth, development, and overall good health.

Vitamins

Vitamins are organic—meaning they come from living matter. Your body needs them to function properly. Vitamin A, the B vitamins ($B_{1, 2, 3, 5, 6, 9}$, and $_{12}$), and vitamins C, D, E, K, and H are the vitamins most often sought by cancer patients.[25]

Because lung cancer and its treatments can affect your appetite and interfere with eating in several ways, your doctor may prescribe supplements. I want to stress how critical it is to <u>TALK TO YOUR DOCTOR FIRST BEFORE TAKING VITAMINS</u>. Fat-soluble vitamins, which the body stores, are toxic in excessive amounts, for example. Some vitamins may adversely affect your treatment, including chemotherapy and surgery, or cause nutritional imbalances. There's even a study suggesting that too many vitamins can give you cancer![26]

Vitamins and their role in lung cancer prevention is an ongoing conversation topic.[27,28] In particular, vitamins with antioxidant activity have received much attention. A number of epidemiological (the study of disease origin and spread) studies have found that beta-carotene may help prevent lung cancer (especially in studies measuring serum concentrations of beta-carotene). The findings from controlled trials, however, contradict this finding, suggesting that people at increased risk, particularly those who smoke, previously smoked, or have worked with asbestos, if given supplementary beta-carotene, might instead be harmed.[29] One study found 18 percent more lung cancers and 8 percent more overall deaths among 29,133 male smokers given a supplement containing 20 mg of beta-carotene and 50 mg of vitamin E.[30] And a recent animal study even found that antioxidants accelerate lung cancer progression.[31]

Although these results don't suggest that beta-carotene supplements cause lung cancer, they do suggest no benefit when smoking or environmental exposure are risk factors. Other studies suggest no positive role for vitamin E, another supplement favored by cancer patients, in lung carcinogenesis.[32] Some epidemiological studies suggest a relationship between increased dietary vitamin C and decreased lung cancer risk, but vitamin C's dietary role is difficult to estimate.[33] A recent meta-analysis of the association between vitamin C intake and lung cancer risk found that "higher intake of vitamin C might have a protective effect against lung cancer" but concluded that a majority of the studies yielded "inconsistent results." It's for these reasons—and many others—that I can't personally endorse antioxidant vitamin supplementation to prevent lung cancer.

Minerals and Trace Elements

Minerals and trace elements are substances that are essential for normal body function. Calcium, iron, magnesium, potassium, fluoride, iodine, and phosphorus are just some of the minerals and trace elements needed for normal body functions. Like vitamins, minerals and trace elements are not manufactured in the body, so we must get them from our food, or supplements, and the amounts of we need of each vary greatly.

A number of minerals and trace elements may play a role in lung cancer prevention or as an adjunctive to more traditional forms of lung cancer therapy.

Calcium Calcium is the most abundant, and certainly one of the human body's most important, minerals. Every one of the body's 37.2 trillion cells contains calcium (a majority of which is found in the bones and teeth). In addition to bone and teeth health, calcium has other important functions, including blood clotting, nerve impulse conduction, muscle contraction, blood pressure, and heart beat regulation. Many foods contain calcium, including dairy products, and cruciferous vegetables, such as broccoli and kale.

Selenium Selenium, found in Brazil nuts, yeast, whole grains, and seafood, is key to healthy immune function, which is especially important for cancer patients. Research has shown that selenium activates an enzyme called glutathione peroxidase, which may help protect the body from cancer. Tests have shown lower than normal levels of selenium in patients with lung cancer. One large study of 1,312 Americans who were treated daily with either selenium or given an inactive substance for 4.5 years and then followed for an additional two years, found a 46 percent decrease in lung cancer incidence and a 53 percent drop in deaths from lung cancer associated with supplemental selenium.[34]

While the evidence appears to show that selenium is important in lung cancer prevention, it is not yet clear whether it can have a beneficial effect after the lung cancer is established.

Zinc You'd quite literally be dead without zinc. Zinc is an element found in more than 300 human enzymes, which speed normal chemical reactions needed in our cells. Immune function, wound repair, tissue growth and other processes depend to some degree on zinc, which comes from dietary sources including meat, eggs, seafood, oysters, black-eyed peas, tofu, and wheat germ.

Some lung cancer patients have been reported to lose excessive amounts of zinc in the urine. In one trial, supplementing such patients with zinc led to an improvement in some aspects of immunity.[35] But the ability, or inability, of zinc supplements to prevent lung cancer or improve survival in those with lung cancer has not been determined.

Other Popular Nutritional Supplements and Products

Many other nutritional supplements are worth mentioning, given their positive role as part of an overall lung cancer treatment program:

Coenzyme Q10 (Ubiquinone)   Coenzymes are substances required by enzymes to propel specific chemical reactions in the body. Coenzyme Q10 (CoQ10) is present in every cell and made naturally by the human body. Coenzymes help enzymes function. Specifically, CoQ10 makes energy needed for the cells to grow and stay healthy. CoQ10 also is a powerful antioxidant—a substance that protects cells from free radical damage. Damaged DNA factors heavily in certain types of cancer. Interestingly, the lowest CoQ10 levels are found in the lungs. CoQ10's role in cancer treatment began more than 50 years ago, when it was found in suboptimal levels in some cancer patients. CoQ10's immune-boosting properties may be helpful for cancer patients and also help cancer from taking root in the first place.

Animal studies looking at CoQ10 have concluded that it does boost immune functioning, helping the body ward off infection and even certain types of cancer. To date, there haven't been any substantive clinical (human) trials involving a sufficient number of patients to determine CoQ10's role in cancer treatment. Clinical trials with small numbers of people have been conducted, but faulty procedure and incomplete information collection resulted in questions regarding whether CoQ10, or something else, was responsible for any benefits reported.[36]

Citrus Pectin   Made from a citrus fruit's peel and pulp, modified citrus pectin (MCP) is easily absorbed by our bodies. An MCP component has been shown in laboratory studies to inhibit cancer cell surface proteins from latching on to new sites or blood vessels. MCP may also inhibit prostate cancer and melanoma (skin cancer) in laboratory animals and cause a reduction in colon tumors in mice. Still, there are no controlled clinical trials to demonstrating MCP's effect on human cancer cells.[37]

Glutamine   Of our body's more than 20 amino acids, glutamine is the most abundant. Glutamine is primarily stored in muscles, but it's also found in the lungs, where, not coincidentally, it's also made. Glutamine removes excess ammonia, supports immune system function, and may be needed for normal brain function and digestion. Our bodies usually make enough glutamine, but many medical conditions, including cancer, lower glutamine levels. Although supplemental glutamine is often given to cancer patients to reduce malnourishment or a chemotherapy-caused diarrhea or inflammation of the mouth called stomatitis, more clinical research is needed to determine whether glutamine is safe or effective as part of any cancer treatment paradigm.[38]

Garlic   Could eating raw garlic help prevent lung cancer? That was the finding published in the respected journal, *Cancer Prevention Research*! A population-based, case-control study carried out over a seven-year period found that people who consumed raw garlic two or more times a week had a 44 percent decreased risk of developing lung cancer. The researchers found a "protective association between intake of raw garlic and lung cancer has been observed with a dose-response pattern, suggesting that garlic may potentially serve as a chemo-preventive agent for lung cancer." Researchers were surprised to find that even among those participants who smoked, eating raw garlic still decreased their risk of lung cancer by around 30 percent.[39]

IP-6   IP-6 (phytic acid and inositol hexaphosphate) is a naturally occurring molecule found in all mammal cells. As an anticancer agent, IP-6 allegedly increases cellular levels of IP-3, an important cell growth and proliferation regulator. Animal and cell studies have shown that IP-6 has anticancer activity, but to date, there have been no studies in people with cancer. Without clinical trial data, it's impossible to know whether IP-6 is an effective anticancer agent.

Melatonin   Melatonin, a hormone made in the pineal gland, is best known for its control of the human sleep cycle, but it may also have a role in cancer prevention and treatment. Melatonin is a powerful antioxidant, scavenging free radicals and regulation antioxidant enzyme levels. Melatonin also affects the immune system, perhaps accounting for its cancer treatment effects in laboratory animals, and it has shown some potential in preliminary human studies.[40] Women with breast cancer have been the most studied group in association with melatonin supplementation,[41] but those studies have been small, so melatonin's role in cancer care remains uncertain.

Noni Juice   Like a number of other fruit-based juices, noni juice contains a host of cancer-fighting nutrients. It's been suggested that chemicals in noni juice may suppress tumor growth by stimulating an immune response. Studies in animal models have shown some support for this theory. However, clinical trials haven't yet been conducted.[42]

Bovine and Shark Cartilage   Cartilage is the tough yet flexible connective tissue found in the skeletons of many animals. Bovine (cow) cartilage and shark cartilage have been studied as a cancer treatment across three decades. It was once thought that sharks, whose skeletons are composed almost entirely of cartilage, didn't get cancer. This is false. Although rare, sharks do get cancer. In the 1970s, scientists reported that bovine cartilage contains a substance that blocks new blood vessel formation. (Cartilage doesn't contain blood vessels, so some wondered if it contained substances that could prevent blood vessel growth around tumors.) Today there is still little scientific evidence that cartilage supplements play an effective role in cancer treatments.

Soy   Powders, milk, capsules, tablets—there seems to be no end to soy's many formulations. Isoflavones are chemicals similar in structure to estrogen, explaining why they're sometimes referred to as "phytoestrogens" or "estrogen mimics." Soybeans and soy products are loaded with isoflavones. Soy's most potent isoflavones, genistein and daidzein, as well as protease inhibitors, phytates, saponins, phytosterols, and lecithin, have powerful effects on the human body. In animal studies, genistein was shown to have anticancer effects, but there are other studies showing a genistein use and an increased cancer risk in genistein- and daidzein-treated animals.[43] Given the controversy surrounding soy and no clear evidence that any benefits outweigh the risks, it might be best for lung cancer patients to avoid soy altogether.

Sun's Soup   "Sun's Soup" and "Selected Vegetables" are herb and vegetable formulations that some claim can fight cancer and help treat a number of other health conditions. Shiitake mushroom, mung bean, *Hedyotis diffusa* (also known by the Chinese herbal name Bai Hua She She Cao), and barbat skullcap (*Scutellaria barbata*; also known by the Chinese herbal name Ban Zhi Lian) all were part of the original Sun soup proprietary formulation. Some Sun's Soup varieties also contain a number of alleged cancer-fighting ingredients, including, scallion, garlic, onion, ginseng, licorice, ginger, olive, and parsley.

According to the National Cancer Institute (NCI), "The use of Selected Vegetables/Sun's Soup as a treatment for human cancer has been investigated in only a limited manner. All available resources . . . [including] the published reports of two clinical studies have identified fewer than 50 treated patients." The NCI went on to say that the results seemed promising, but with such a small number (27 total) of patients treated, it was not possible to draw overall conclusions. The NCI recommends that "[a]dditional larger, well-designed clinical studies that test identical formulations of vegetables and herbs are necessary to determine more clearly whether Selected Vegetables/Sun's Soup can be useful in the treatment of non–small cell lung and other types of cancer."[44]

Can Bone Broth Heal Cancer?

You've probably read a number of stories about bone broth and its promise of readily absorbable, super nutrition. Restaurants from New York to Los Angeles are offering it and there's even a best-selling bone broth book.

Bone broth isn't new. People have been dumping every animal part imaginable into pots to make rich, nourishing broths for hundreds of years. How do you think chicken soup got its nickname "Jewish penicillin"?

What concerns me is that the list of bone broth's magical healing and restorative properties is getting longer by the day. As with so many proposed cures in the alternative/integrative medicine realm, there are few scientific studies expounding bone broth's healthful properties. As noted health journalist Amy Blaszyk observed in an NPR story, "There is no one bone broth recipe. It can be made with different animal bones (some with fatty marrow, some without), with different added flavors (like onions and herbs) and with different cooking methods (five hours of simmering versus 24 hours or more). All of those variables impact the nutritional properties and will give you a different broth."[45]

Additionally, some of the scientific claims bone broth aficionados make are just flat-out wrong. One popular book says that bone broth is a "gelatin-rich liquid that provides the amino acids necessary to make collagen," which, among other things, builds bone structure.

We don't absorb whole collagen, so the idea that eating it will somehow promote bone growth falls into the realm of magical thinking. Moreover, as the broth cooks, its disease-fighting vitamins and enzymes get denatured from heat, rendering them less useful.

On the other hand, chicken broth, aka chicken soup, may boost immune health. A study published in the journal *Chest* found that people with an upper respiratory tract infection ate chicken soup, showed slightly lower inflammatory response, possibly as a result of carnosine, a compound in chicken soup, that inhibits reaction to the infection by the neutrophils, a type of white blood cell. In the study, carnosine both inhibited inflammation and prevented the virus from replicating.[46]

By no means does this mean that the immune-boosting properties of chicken soup can help fight off cancer. Where broth can be of benefit to cancer patients is in replacing nutrients, including sodium, lost during treatment. Broth may also provide amino acids needed to rebuild weak, atrophied muscle.

My advice: Don't be deluded into thinking that one magic food or group of foods can rid you of cancer. We've been down this road before. Two years ago, juicing was all the rage. Now it's been discredited.[47] Bone broth can be part of a nutritionally balanced diet, which is critical for cancer patients, but there's little evidence to suggest not a "super food" or "miracle food source" that can cure what ails us, including cancer.

Herbs and Botanicals

Alternative medicines, including homeopathy, Chinese medicine, and Ayurveda incorporate herbs and botanicals—dried mixtures of plants or plant parts that are dispensed loose or given in pill or capsule form.

Following is a brief review of some common herbs and botanicals used by cancer patients.

Astragalus

Astragalus membranaceus, or astragalus, has been a Chinese medicine mainstay for thousands of years (see below). Astragalus proponents believe the herb's dried root increases immune system activity, strength, and wound healing. Some studies suggest astragalus may have antitumor effects, specifically against melanoma and leukemia.[48] And limited animal studies seem to support astragalus' immune-enhancing effects. A small clinical trial by Chinese researchers found that an astragalus-based compound commonly used in traditional Chinese medicine improved quality of life for patients with advanced non–small cell lung cancer.[49] There are no large-scale studies looking at astragalus as an adjuvant for lung cancer treatment, however.[50]

Chinese Herbal Remedies

Traditional Chinese medicine is popular among cancer patients, but the consumer should be aware there are potential side effects. Studies have not been large or sufficiently well designed to provide thorough evidence, and herbal remedies can contain a number of contaminants.

Practitioners dispense herb mixtures chosen for a patient's particular needs.* With TCM now so sought-after by consumers, many TCM professionals have started selling and marketing preset herbal therapies. Unfortunately, there have been more than a few instances where these formulas didn't deliver what was promised. Indeed, quantity and quality are in short supply in many herbal remedies. New York–based consumerlab.com, a company that tests, rates, and reviews such products, found that many herbal remedies contain contaminants, including prescription drugs, toxins, and microbes. I suspect that few manufacturers of herbal medicine products adhere to scrupulous production practices.

A 2013 review of 24 Chinese clinical trials on non–small cell lung cancer concluded that, when used in combination with other therapies, Chinese herbal remedies might reduce the toxicity of chemotherapy, increase tumor response to treatment, and increase survival rates. The review also noted improvement on the Karnofsky

---

Never take any herbs, botanicals, or other supplements without first speaking with your cancer care providers. Many can have unexpected side effects, especially if you are receiving traditional medications, chemotherapy, or radiation.

Performance Status scale, which reflects patients' functional impairment, in some individuals. But it also noted that there were no large-scale trials that were randomized and thus capable of showing wide effects that could be attributed with certainty to the herb use and not to other factors. So, again, it is wisest to consider herbs with caution. Some herbs may interfere with treatment or cause potentially dangerous side effects. Herbs may seem harmless, but as I've said before, if they're powerful enough to heal, they're powerful enough to harm.[51]

Essiac Tea

Essiac tea is an herbal mixture that has not been tested in clinical trials, so there is no scientific evidence regarding its effects. Proponents claim it leads to mass reduction in tumors by strengthening immune system function, reduces pain, and increases survival rates.[52] Essiac tea contains plant parts, including burdock root (*Arctium lappa*), slippery elm bark (*Ulmus fulva*), sheep sorrel (*Rumex acetosella*), and Turkish or Indian rhubarb (*Rheum palmatum* or *Rheum officianale*). Burdock root has been shown to inhibit development of cancer in laboratory animals and rhubarb extract has shown anticancer activity in nonhuman lab tests.[53,54]

Green Tea

Green tea is a Chinese tea variety that comes from the *Camellia sinensis* plant. Green tea famously contains polyphenols, chemicals that act as antioxidants, and catechins, polyphenol compounds that are valued for their anticancer properties, alkaloids, and amino acids (among other ingredients). Epigallocatechin-3-gallate (EGCG) is green tea's most active and abundant catechin. Because EGCG, along with ECG (epicatechin gallate), is a free radical scavenger, it may protect cells from DNA damage, making it a potentially useful as a component of cancer treatment.[55] Tea polyphenols have also been shown to block tumor cell spread and encourage apoptosis in laboratory and animal studies.[56] Green tea catechins also have been shown to inhibit angiogenesis and tumor cell invasiveness and to activate enzymes that may protect against tumor development.[57]

Licorice

Known also as gan cao, the licorice plant's dried root has been a Chinese medicine mainstay for thousands of years. Some early studies indicate glycyrrhizin, the main active ingredient in the licorice root, might have protective properties against liver cancer. However, efforts to establish glycyrrhizin's cancer-fighting promise went down the drain after long-term consumption led to high blood pressure and even swelling of the brain in some patients.[58] Another licorice ingredient, isoangustone A, may provide same benefits as glycyrrhizin without the side effects and is being studied with malignant melanoma patients.[59]

Milk Thistle

In some circles, milk thistle has been hailed for the chemical silymarin, as laboratory experiments have determined it has potent antioxidant effects and has been shown to hinder the growth of some cancer cells in laboratory experiments including prostate, skin, and breast cancers.[60] However, this effect has yet to be demonstrated with humans because there have been no clinical studies.

Turmeric

Turmeric root is a Chinese and ayurvedic medicine mainstay. It's also a spice that has been used in cooking for centuries. Other common names for turmeric include Indian saffron, Indian valerian, jiang huang, radix, and red valerian. Turmeric is from the plant *Curcuma longa*, the root of which is used both as a spice and as a medicine. Turmeric's health effects are linked to the compound curcumin. Both tumeric and curcumin are alleged to have strong tumor-inhibiting properties, stemming from the plant's antioxidant properties, which lead to a number of metabolic actions in cancer cells.[61] An average turmeric root only contains, at best, 5 percent curcumin, and powdered turmeric root is not controlled to be standardized; thus, an undetermined but certainly very large amount of the product would be needed to see any tangible benefit. Curcumin is also poorly absorbed from the gastrointestinal tract, meaning it has low bioavailability.

In one study, tumeric-protected rats exposed to known carcinogens were protected from colon, stomach, and skin cancers.[62] In laboratory studies, turmeric also stopped tumor cell replication, but it's unknown whether this effect occurs in the human body. Positive results have been shown in pancreatic cancer patients, and there are ongoing studies looking at curcumin's effectiveness as an adjuvant cancer treatment. Other studies, however, have suggested that dietary curcumin might interfere with some chemotherapy drugs, so great caution must be exercised when using curcumin.[63]

Can Spicing Up Your Meals Help You Fight Cancer?

The news is in, and it looks promising! Eating spicy food every day lowers the risk of early death from cancer and other serious health ailments. One large study including almost 500,000 Chinese people between ages 30 and 79 showed that those who ate a spicy meal regularly—at least every other day—were less likely to die of cancer than those who only ate a spicy meal less than once a week. Those who ate spicy meals more often were 14 percent less likely to die of cancer. The strongest links in death reduction were associated with lower rates of death from cancer, heart disease, and breathing disorders. The lower death rates were most clear in frequent spicy meal eaters who did not drink alcohol.

It should be noted that the study could not draw any concrete conclusions about the effects of a spicy diet and absolute causes of lower death rates in those who often eat them, because the study looked only at the broad statistical outcomes and did not determine what specific role spices might have played in the apparent better health. In summation, the study showed a correlation between the two but did not explore or prove causation.

Earlier studies determined a similar correlation between a specific spicy food—chili peppers—and health benefits. It is suspected that a natural element in chili peppers, capsaicin, may help prevent cancer, obesity, and inflammation, as well as other disorders and diseases. The study's authors noted that Chinese people generally have a different diet and lifestyle from Westerners, and those differences may also play a role, or contribute to, the health reactions seen with frequent eaters of spicy meals.

So, enjoy your spicy food, but don't expect a miracle.[64]

Acupuncture and Related Therapies

Given its steadily growing popularity, it's hard to believe that acupuncture is actually a 5,000-year-old practice. Like other alternative medicine practices, acupuncture is based on qi, or energy flow through the body, along paths known as meridians. Acupuncturists insert fine needles at particular points along the meridians, aiming to restore the energy flow, thus relieving pain and treating disease and/or side effects. A session may include the use of heat, provided by burning the herb mugwort, during acupuncture. Acupressure, or tui na, is a form of massage therapy that involves manipulation of the same acupuncture points. Cupping, as the name implies, is an additional acupuncture-based treatment that works by applying cups to the acupuncture points. Cupping causes blood to pool at the cupped site, so it may be traumatic for those new to the discipline.

Anecdotal reports suggest that many cancer-related symptoms and treatment side effects such as chronic pain, nausea and vomiting, anxiety, and depression are helped with acupuncture. Limited studies demonstrating acupuncture's efficacy were convincing enough for the National Institutes of Health to state that "acupuncture is a proven effective treatment modality for nausea and vomiting."[65] Acupuncture has also been used to treat constipation, diarrhea, and loss of appetite. The jury is still out when it comes to acupuncture's effectiveness in treating other common cancer-related symptoms, such as diarrhea.

The National Comprehensive Cancer Network guidelines for adult cancer pain recommend acupuncture as one of several integrative interventions that can be used in conjunction with pharmacologic intervention. Postoperative cancer pain, postoperative nausea and vomiting, postsurgical gastroparesis syndrome, opioid-induced constipation, opioid-induced pruritus, chemotherapy-induced neuropathy, aromatase inhibitor–associated joint pain, and neck dissection–related pain and dysfunction are all thought to be helped with acupuncture.

Aside from anecdotes—reports from patients—there is also some experimental evidence showing that cancer patients have better immune system function, after acupuncture but no published studies have proven such immune system changes resulting from acupuncture alter the disease's progression or patients' survival rates.

Pulling It All Together

Health and disease are part of a continuum that includes a person's physical, mental, spiritual, and social well-being. Thus, those of us on the frontlines in the war against cancer should consider whether our patients would benefit from a holistic treatment approach—one that addresses all dimensions of human well-being. In this chapter, we learned that there are a number of approaches to optimizing our health. Allopathic medicine may always serve as the foundation for cancer treatment. However, used wisely and with proper guidance, other disciplines could become a cornerstone of future cancer treatments.

Whatever you decide, please discuss any treatment decisions with <u>your doctor and other cancer care team members</u> to ensure the safety and effectiveness of your approach. My hope is that your life, and the lives of all of your loved ones, friends, and associates who may face or be struggling with cancer, are bettered by having this information.

Step IV
Ask the Right Questions

CHAPTER 7

Managing Your Lung Cancer Care

Takeaways

- In the age of the Affordable Care Act, you have a right to quality health care, regardless of your current circumstances, including a cancer diagnosis.
- Take a proactive role in the treatment and management of your illness. This is all about empowerment, which can offer you a sense of control during a time of great uncertainty.
- Self-advocacy doesn't mean you have to fly solo. Self-advocacy, in fact, means seeking added support from friends, family members, and health care professionals.
- Don't be afraid to ask your doctor and other health care providers questions.
- Cancer.net, National Cancer Institute, and the Lung Cancer Alliance offer a number of e-sources for lung cancer patients, including lists of organizations, programs, services, and support for patients and their families.
- Counseling, patient navigation services, support groups, nutritional guidance, and fitness classes are some of the services offered at your hospital or clinic. Take advantage of them.
- Connect to other lung cancer patients. Shared experiences, especially those involving hardship, are a powerful healing tool.
- Seek a second opinion about your diagnosis or treatment plan.
- Even with health insurance, cancer care is expensive. Ask for help managing nonmedical issues, and finances, in particular.
- Find ways to communicate your needs, know your options, and understand the doctor's opinion, and express your preferences.

Introduction

Even people with health insurance are probably unfamiliar with the internal workings of the Byzantine U.S. health care system. While the Affordable Care Act (ACA) has provided access to quality health services for millions of uninsured Americans, it has also created a fair share of confusion. As William W. Stead, chief information officer at Vanderbilt University Medical Center, said in a recent study, "[The] current healthcare environment is characterized by competition, misaligned incentives, and inherent distrust among stakeholders."[1]

This chapter attempts to end some of the distrust and confusion. It offers basic information about the U.S. health care system in the wake of the ACA and 2015 Supreme Court ruling, so you can use this information to get the best possible health care. Read, consider your choices, and ask questions of those professionals who play any role in your lung cancer care.

Step 1: Become an Informed Health Care Consumer

The U.S. health care system is a big business. Under the Affordable Care Act, it has also morphed into an enormous, cumbersome bureaucracy with rules and regulations that change almost daily. Even several years after it became the law of the land, the ACA still puzzles people. A survey in the respected *Consumer Reports* found that 36 percent of people believe that the ACA allows the government to determine which doctor they can see.[2] This is false, but the public's perception is not surprising. A study in the journal *Health Affairs* reported that just 60 percent of people understand key concepts related to insurance, such as co-pays, deductibles, premiums, and provider networks.[3] Still, the ACA is here to stay and has produced some positive results, including a significant reduction in the rate of the nation's uninsured.

For many of my patients, the ACA put an end to years of playing health care musical chairs. Gone were the days of leapfrogging from one insurance plan to another, and haggling over services, especially if they switched jobs, or were unemployed for any significant amount of time. But signing up for the ACA—which includes wading through a blur of numbers indicating various premiums, copays, and deductibles—isn't easy, even with proper guidance. Certainly, there's also a fair segment of the population that doesn't appreciate having to pay a penalty for not having health insurance or would be shocked to learn that they might have to pay back a portion of the government subsidies they received to offset the onerous cost of insurance.

Also, compared with the average workplace employee, anyone purchasing health insurance through government exchanges encounters a whole different set of challenges. Finding the right coverage is especially complex for those receiving government subsidies because they're required to estimate their annual income, which isn't always predictable.

Other problems occur at the state and local level, especially in places where the local government isn't fully on board and doesn't support the law. In Texas, where former governor Rick Perry decried passage of the ACA as a "criminal act," information isn't always widely available and is seldom clear.

If you have lung cancer, politics aren't part of your day-to-day reality. You're a health care consumer. You need information. You need quality, affordable health care. And you need these things now. To make informed, wise decisions, you first have to know what you need, and, second, know how to get it. Even for a person in perfect health and with unlimited financial resources, this isn't an easy task. It's even more complicated when you toss in a life-altering illness like lung cancer. Lung cancer doesn't care whether you call Park Avenue or the North Pole home.

In 2016, the information stream courses nonstop through the public sphere. You're both a lung cancer patient and a health care consumer. Thus, it's your job to get informed about how the law works and how it affects you. Don't wait for someone to show you the way.

Self-education is the first and most important step in dealing with information overload. You're more likely to find optimal health care that suits your personality and preferences, not to mention budget, if you're knowledgeable about your condition, the health care system, and your consumer rights.

Although I wish you'd never been diagnosed with lung cancer, there are times when the biggest obstacles turn into the greatest opportunities. As a lung cancer patient, you will enter a new realm of language, experiences, people, and friends. This realm, including, perhaps first-time exposure to the complexity of the American health care system, could at first seem overwhelming. But like anything else, as you familiarize yourself with its policies and procedures, the road ahead becomes clearer. And I am certain you will shortly find that road.

Gathering Information

All lung cancer patients must take an active role in securing quality health care. Seek information and educate yourself. For most patients, lung cancer wasn't even on the radar before diagnosis. Now things will never be the same. Learn about lung cancer to gain a measure of control over your situation, make better-informed treatment decisions, understand and manage your symptoms, and plan wisely for the future. The more you know about your disease, the less confused and anxious you'll feel as you embark on your journey. Simply picking up this book is an important first step in the self-education process.

Who's on First: Your Cancer Care Team

It seems obvious, but the best place to start gathering information is right from the horse's mouth. Few people will be as intimately familiar with you and have a better sense of your needs than your lung cancer team. Below are some of the most frequently asked questions and comments I hear from cancer patients. You may want to ask your lung cancer team members the very same questions. Don't be embarrassed. Outside of experts in medicine and bioscience, few people—even those with PhDs in other fields—know the answers. If you have a question, regardless of how seemingly simple or complicated it is, ask it. The only dumb question is the one that is not asked.

Common Questions and Comments from Lung Cancer Patients

- How did I get sick?
- Are you sure I have lung cancer? Maybe you missed something.
- What type of lung cancer do I have, and why does it matter?
- How advanced (what stage) is my disease?
- Am I going to die?
- Will my health insurance cover the cost of treatment?
- What are the best treatment options?
- What treatments do you recommend?
- What will happen if I don't follow your recommendations?
- What are the risks or side effects associated with the treatment(s) you are recommending?
- Do I have any other options? What about alternative treatments?
- What are the benefits of the other treatments? What are the possible risks and side effects?
- I read online of a popular treatment for lung cancer treatment that's only available in Europe. What do you think of this treatment?

- What are clinical trials? Are there clinical trials that might be right for my condition?

I hear other comments and questions, of course, but I think you get the picture. View every appointment with your doctor or other health care professional as an opportunity to get answers to any questions you may have. Stop thinking that your questions are "stupid" or "trivial" or that you're wasting the doctor's valuable time. We're talking about your life.

Since you'll likely have a number of questions for your doctor or health care provider, consider writing them down before your appointment. This will help you organize your thoughts and prioritize your questions. Your doctor wants to help you, and doctors cannot do that fully if they do not know your questions and concerns. And there may be something on the list that's more important than you realized—a problem requiring immediate attention.

National Cancer Institute

The National Cancer Institute (www.nci.nih.gov) is one of the best public resources for A-to-Z lung cancer information. Here, you'll find everything you need to know about lung cancer, including diagnosis, staging, treatment, coping with cancer, clinical trials, nutrition, and support groups. On the NCI website you'll find the Physician Data Query (PDQ), a massive database containing the most-up-to-date information about lung cancer treatment, screening, prevention, and psychological and supportive care. You can access the same information offered on the NCI site via Cancer Information Service at: www.cissecure.nci.nih.gov/ncipubs.

Additional Resources

If you can get past the technical jargon and multisyllabic words—no easy feat—medical journal articles feature up-to-date, scientifically sound information on lung cancer research and treatments. Jennifer Raff is a professor of biological anthropology at the University of Kansas. She's written an informative, not to mention entertaining, blog on how to read and understand a scientific paper. You'll find it at: http://violentmetaphors.com/2013/08/25/how-to-read-and-under stand-a-scientific-paper-2/.

Cancer education pamphlets, online materials that can be printed or downloaded, teleconferences, and live online lectures are some of the free products and services available through the nonprofit CancerCare. For more information, check out the organization's website at: http://www.cancercare.org.

Founded in 1995 by lung cancer survivor Peggy McCarthy, the Lung Cancer Alliance is the oldest and only national nonprofit lung cancer patient advocacy and support organization. The Lung Cancer Alliance website contains some of the most up-to-date lung cancer information you'll find anywhere. Information about all things lung cancer, including available treatments, prevention, clinical trials, exciting research, and support services can be found at http://www .lungcanceralliance.org.

There are many other lung cancer–centric books, websites, blogs, and organizations listed in this book's resource section.

Patients' Rights

Growing up on suburban Long Island just outside New York City, I remember a television commercial for a popular clothing store that always concluded with the tagline "An educated consumer is our best customer." To be an educated lung cancer consumer, first and foremost, you need to know your patient rights and the rules of conduct between patients and medical caregivers (as well as the institutions that support them). I want to empower you, the health care consumer, to self-advocate so you receive the very best cancer care. Whether you have the most expensive private health insurance, purchased your coverage through the ACA, or receive Medicaid, you're entitled to the very best care.

In November 1997, President Bill Clinton established the Advisory Commission on Consumer Protection and Quality, which, in one of its first official acts, issued the first Patient Bill of Rights and Responsibilities. There's a threefold goal to this bill:

- To strengthen consumer confidence that the U.S. health care system is fair and meets consumer needs and to ensure that patients take a proactive role in getting and staying healthy
- To stress the importance of a strong relationship between patients and their health care providers
- To reaffirm the critical role consumers play in safeguarding their own health

The Advisory Commission's recommendations were not legally binding, but they did represent the collective wisdom of our country's leading health care stakeholders. For more information, visit: www .cancer.org/treatment/findingandpayingfortreatment/understanding financialandlegalmatters/patients-bill-of-rights.

The Dream Team: Your Cancer Care Professionals

"Dreams take teams," a friend used to tell me, and it's certainly true. No one can go it alone, especially when it comes to lung cancer. Quality cancer care requires a dedicated, expert, multidisciplinary team. Depending on the disease stage, your team may include some or all of the following health care professionals.[4]

- Dietician/Nutritionist—A person who will help determine your dietary needs and plan your meals.
- Dosimetrist—A person who determines proper radiation treatment dosage.
- Medical Oncologist—A physician specializing in the nonsurgical treatment of benign and malignant tumors.
- Thoracic Surgeon—A doctor who operates on conditions involving the chest.
- Pathologist—A doctor who studies the cause and development of disease.
- Primary Care Provider/General Practitioner—Medical professional responsible for your overall care and can include any number of practitioners, including an internist or gynecologist.
- Oncology Nurse—A nurse specializing in the care and treatment of cancer patients.
- Pulmonologist—A doctor who specializes in diagnosing and treating noncancerous lung disorders, and frequently a physician who first diagnoses lung cancer.[5]
- Radiation Oncologist—A doctor who uses radiation therapy to treat cancer; similar to a radiologist who uses X-rays and other forms of radiation to diagnose and treat disease.
- Psychiatric Social Worker (PSW)/Psychologist or Psychiatrist—I advise patients to find someone specifically trained to deal with cancer's emotional wallop. PSWs, for example, can point cancer patients in the direction of the appropriate medical, social, financial, and supportive services.[6]
- Oncology Advance Practice Nurse (APN)—A specialist nurse who has advanced education and training in cancer treatment.

Finding the Right Stuff: Physician Qualifications

You have a say in choosing your health care providers. This is critically important because your cancer care team will help you make life-changing decisions. All cancer patients require a certain comfort level with the cancer care team and must feel confident about the quality of care they provide. Your team, not to mention the facilities where you'll receive treatment, bears directly on treatment outcome. Highly skilled and experienced cancer care professionals can make all the difference.

Medical Licensure   It may seem obvious, but physicians must be duly licensed to practice medicine in their respective states. States have their own unique licensing requirements. Call your state licensing board or visit http://www.ama-assn.org/ama/pub/education-careers /becoming-physician/medi cal-licensure/state-medical-boards.page to see if your doctor is on the up and up.

Board Certification   After residency training, doctors typically become board-certified in their respective specialties. Independent specialty boards (unaffiliated with state medical licensing agencies) certify doctors once they meet specific requirements, which include a valid medical license, specific educational and training criteria, and proof of passing a specialty board examination, the contents of which are determined by the independent specialty board. American Board of Medical Specialties (ABMS) and the American Medical Association (AMA) recognizes 24 specialty boards and a number of subspecialty boards. Subspecialty eligibility is based on umbrella specialty certification. ABMS boards of interest to people with lung cancer include but aren't limited to:

- American Board of Internal Medicine; subspecialties include:
  - Medical Oncology
  - Pulmonary Diseases
- American Board of Pathology
- American Board of Radiology; subspecialties include:
  - Diagnostic Radiology
  - Radiation Oncology
  - Radiologic Physics
- American Board of Surgery
- American Board of Thoracic Surgery
- American Board of Anesthesiology; subspecialties include:

- Pain Medicine
- Hospice and Palliative Medicine

Visit   http://www.abms.org/member-boards/specialty-subspecialty
-certificates/ and https://www.certificationmatters.org/is-your-doctor
-board-certified/search-now.aspx for more information.

Professional Medical Society Membership   Medical society membership is another important feather in the cap for doctors. Professional
medical societies for physicians involved in the treatment of lung
cancer include:

- American College of Chest Physicians
- American College of Radiology
- American College of Surgeons
- American Society of Clinical Oncology
- American Society of Clinical Pathologists
- American Society of Internal Medicine
- College of American Pathologists
- Radiological Society of North America
- Society of Thoracic Surgery

The Doctor Will See You Now

A medical oncologist is often the first cancer care team member selected, although he or she typically comes by referral from an internist,
surgeon, pulmonologist, or insurance provider. Query other lung cancer patients, especially long-term survivors, for a referral as well. From
there, the oncologist can refer you to the other players you'll need to
fill your roster. If the professional you're speaking with seems uncomfortable, vague, or unenthusiastic about another health care professional, suspect that where there's smoke there's also fire. Consider
moving on to another health care professional. Hospitals and local
medical societies have patient referral services. There are a number of
other resources for finding doctors to treat your lung cancer.

Rounding Out Your Cancer Care Team

Dreams need teams. Beating lung cancer requires a team of expert
health care professionals, each with specialized training and expertise.
While a doctor might quarterback your team, it's the allied health

professionals (nonphysician) with whom you'll interact most often and who see to your day-to-day care.

The Patient–Doctor Partnership

Lung cancer is a life-altering illness. People living with the disease make life-changing decisions almost daily. Decision making is an art, a skill unique to each of us. Some of my patients are information junkies who don't give a second thought to spending hours trolling the Internet in search of the latest lung cancer findings. These people are independent thinkers, preferring, for the most part, their own counsel and relying lightly on physician guidance. And I'll be perfectly honest: There are more than a handful doctors who won't accept a backseat role.

Other patients—the majority, from my experience—give it all away. They willingly cede control, believing that someone with more knowledge, experience, and expertise should take the reins in the decision-making process. "Too many cooks spoil the broth," is how one patient put it. At the risk of playing both sides of the fence, I'll admit there are no easy answers. There are pros and cons to all patient–doctor partnerships. I'd like to say that optimal cancer care occupies a middle ground. It's an equal partnership, or at least it should be. But I'll admit there is a fair percentage of people who do better with one extreme or the other. There's really no special algorithm or magic formula for choosing the best treatment path. I tell patients, "Find what's best for you and your life."

Do we shape our own destiny, or are we fate's unwilling pawns? How much control do we ultimately have over the course of our lives? These are some of the many questions cancer patients ask themselves following a positive diagnosis. I get it. We all want to have a say in shaping our own destinies. Cancer strips us of any illusion that we might be in control of our lives. Anger, fear, resignation or sadness—these are just a few of the intense emotions experienced by cancer patients following a positive diagnosis. Having a say in the treatment process can restore some this control.

Circumstances will also factor heavily in your decision making. Patients facing surgery will almost certainly defer to a doctor, even if that means seeking a second opinion. But some decisions, such as eating better, exercising more, and reducing stress can be made independent of a doctor. Bottom line: You're going to need support no matter what, so find people who complement your personality and decision-making style.

Talking the Talk

Clear and open communication is critical for any relationship, especially the one between doctor and patient, so I've highlighted the five most critical components of quality cancer care.

1. Be open and honest with your doctor about any topic that may come up.
2. Never be afraid or embarrassed to ask questions if you feel unsure or don't understand something.
3. Demonstrate respect for, and politely demand the respect of, your health care providers. Just because you wear a white coat doesn't mean you know how to talk to people.
4. As the relationship evolves, bring up issues that are bound to arise.
5. Don't be afraid to respectfully question your health care provider's decision making and even seek a second opinion if you're unsatisfied with an answer you receive. Just be sure to question mindfully. Always listen to your inner voice if something doesn't make sense.

Most patients only feel comfortable speaking with their doctor privately. Don't be shy about telling your doctor about your need for privacy and about any information that should be kept private.

If you've given someone Power of Attorney, provide your doctors, or other relevant personnel, with a copy of your Advance Directive and Power of Attorney documents. You should also designate a trusted loved one or friend as someone the doctor can speak to about your health care needs and treatment if you ever are unable to speak or advocate for yourself. For many people, that person is a spouse, sibling, or adult child. Be sure your doctor's office is aware of this person and knows how to contact him or her. There may be a need to put in writing that the person has your permission to advocate on your behalf if you ever cannot do so yourself.

Working It Out: Breaking Through Communication Difficulties

All human relationships have their tough times and upsets. The relationships with your cancer team members are no different. Negative feelings can hinder the effectiveness of this critical relationship. If you find yourself becoming angry with your doctor, don't hurl invectives, make caustic remarks, or ask questions that put your provider on the defensive or make him or her feel slighted or marginalized. There will be many days when you're feeling lousy, sad, or stressed. Your doctor will have these days too, and you may not realize it. All of this influences the nature and quality of patient–doctor interactions. How could it not? But patient–doctor tension always affects patient care so it's important to work through rough patches early. If something is troubling you, speak up or send the doctor an e-mail. Nothing should interfere with your peace of mind or treatment.

Should I Seek a Second Opinion?

What if you can't work through your differences, best efforts notwithstanding? We've all heard of second opinions. Some health plans even require a second opinion. Find another doctor, because even if you ultimately decide to stay put, there's nothing wrong with soliciting a different point of view. If you decide to leave, your current doctor should continue providing care until you find a replacement.

You may be able to appeal the second-opinion requirement. Check with your insurance company to determine how you can do that and what forms are needed.

Choosing a Treatment Facility

This is one of most difficult decisions facing lung cancer patients. Often, patient are directed to a particular hospital or treatment center because their doctor is affiliated with that facility. Your insurance plan, especially if you have Medicaid or some other low-cost plan, also factors in. People living in rural communities in particular may have few options within a reasonable traveling distance.

Types of Cancer Care Facilities

Community Hospitals Community hospitals, university-affiliated teaching hospitals, and cancer centers all provide optimal cancer care. For people living in rural areas or at a great distance from a major medical center, or for those who simply like the idea of being treated close to home, community hospitals are an important resource. Some patients prefer a smaller, more personalized setting, don't want to be inconvenienced or incur additional expenses, or may not be well enough to travel long distances. Some local hospitals may have limited experience with certain procedures or may lack access to the newest medical equipment, so research is needed before going this route. Regardless of facility size, I counsel patients to find a facility that has extensive experience treating lung cancer patients and one that offers a comprehensive team approach to treating their illness.

Teaching and University-Affiliated Hospitals   A teaching hospital or university-affiliated hospital is an academic medical center, meaning it's a medical school–affiliated facility. As the name implies, these hospitals are equally committed to patient care and educational activities, as they provide training to medical students, nurses, postgraduate fellows, and other health care professionals. Many are renowned for their clinical research programs, which have the resources to fund state-of-the-art facilities. Drugs, medical devices, and new treatment methods are developed and tested at these facilities, explaining why they're frequently the facility of choice for cancer patients. There are more than 1,000 teaching hospitals in the United States, so even those living in rural areas can probably find a facility not too far from home.

Urbanites, or anyone living near a city, can seek out an NCI-supported cancer center. There are 69 NCI-affiliated cancer centers spread across 35 states and the District of Columbia. There are literally hundreds of clinical trials under way at these centers. These centers frequently partner with other facilities. The majority of these facilities are university affiliated, although some are research-only facilities. There are three types of facilities:

- The NCI supports seven **Basic Laboratory Cancer Centers,** which conduct only laboratory research and don't treat patients.
- The NCI's 45 **Comprehensive Cancer Centers** conduct basic science, offer clinical services, and prevention and control research. These centers also offer community outreach and cancer education programs.
- Seventeen **Clinical Cancer Centers** conduct clinical (patient-based) research and may have other research programs.

You can get more information about NCI cancer program at http://www.cancer.gov/research/nci-role/cancer-centers.

There are also community-based cancer care centers and oncology outpatient facilities offering specialized cancer care. The American

College of Surgeons Commission on Cancer provides standards and guidelines for community cancer center programs and and for accreditation process.

The Joint Commission (JC), an independent, nonprofit organization accredits and certifies more than 20,000 health care organizations and programs, inspecting hospitals and healthcare facilities to ensure they meet JC quality standards. JC accreditation is not required for a facility to operate, but the organization's stamp of approval is a good indication that a facility meets high standards.

The Hospital: How to Choose

Finding the best hospital for the treatment you need means learning as much as you can about the hospital's quality of care. Like any other businesses, some hospitals offer higher quality. Research has shown, for example, that hospitals that most often perform a particular type of surgery usually boast a better outcome for patients that need that surgery.

Questions You Should Ask When Choosing a Cancer Care Hospital

1. Does the hospital meet national quality standards?
2. How do the patient outcomes (surgery and recovery results) at one hospital compare with the results at others nearby?
3. Does my doctor have privileges (permission to admit patients) at the hospital?
4. Does the hospital accept my health insurance plan?
5. Does the hospital have experience treating lung cancer?
6. Has the hospital successfully treated lung cancer?

Dr. Presser's Quick Tips for Finding a Quality Hospital

- The hospital has proper accreditation.
- The hospital has been rated by independent state, consumer, or other trusted groups.
- Your doctor has privileges there.
- The hospital accepts multiple health plans.
- The hospital specializes in treating your cancer type and has successfully treated or routinely treats your type of cancer.

Your Hospital Experience

Hospitals and lung cancer patients go hand in hand, like flip sides of the same coin. A hospital is a world unto itself, with its own culture, customs, and language. If you've ever been hospitalized, you know that it can be a challenging experience, even under the best of circumstances. Hospital staffs, especially in cities, are busy, pressed for time, and preoccupied with the bottom line—getting patients in and out the door. They're also frequently understaffed and overworked. They have patient needs to meet and don't have time to respond to every little whim or feeling. It's depersonalizing, not to mention depressing, to be considered in terms of your disease, rather than your name, but it happens.

"I felt like an object, not a person," said a patient after receiving the depersonalized "disease" designation. Any facility caring for thousands of people at any given time will have procedures and process that must follow so that everything runs smoothly. Patients must fit the mold; few facilities will construct the mold around them. It's just not possible to do otherwise. Additionally, hospital personnel, particularly in large, heavily populated urban areas, are stressed beyond belief, and frequently given more responsibilities than they can reasonably handle. As a cancer patient, you must juggle two competing realities: your need—and right—to get the best care possible versus the reality of a large hospital culture. My only suggestion is that you express your needs but do it politely. Build a positive relationship with the hospital staff. Don't come off as rude, demanding, or unreasonable. A hospital staff that's treated with respect and consideration will respond in turn.

To optimize your hospital experience, try the following approaches.

- **Be Strategic.**
  Find out who will be supervising your care and how to reach this person before, during, and even after your hospital stay. Ask the supervising physician who else will be involved in your care.
- **Build Bridges.**
  Be honest and kind to the hospital staff. Let them know you appreciate what they do for you. You probably know from your own life that people who feel appreciated are generally more willing to lend a helping hand.

- **Ask Questions.**
  Don't be a shrinking violet. Don't be the proverbial fly on the wall. If you want to know something, ask. Most hospital staff members want to help. Give them the opportunity.

Supplemental Care Services

Lung cancer patients can avail themselves of a number of health care and ancillary services. You can find additional information about these services in this book's resource section or on any of the websites listed in this chapter.

Home Health Care   Home health care is an option for cancer patients that, in many instances, offers the same services as a hospital or outpatient facility, including intravenous (IV) therapy such as chemotherapy infusions, supplemental fluids, and antibiotics; blood draws for laboratory tests; physical therapy; and home health aides. Coverage for home health care services varies from one health insurance provider and plan to another. Check with your insurance provider to see what, if any, coverage you have for these services. The American Cancer Society offers a complete breakdown of home health care, including a list of agencies providing such services, on its website at http://www.cancer.org/treatment/findingandpaying fortreatment/choosingyourtreatmentteam/homecareagencies/home -care-agencies-toc.

Some states provide payments to the primary caregivers of seriously ill patients. Contact your state health department or the Patient Advocate Foundation at 800-532-5274 to find out if financial support is available. You can also search the state resource guide available on the Patient Advocate Foundation website at http://www .patientadvocate.org/index.php.

Hospice   Lung cancer, and all cancer for that matter, is a serious illness, one that, despite recent breakthroughs, some people don't survive. Hospice care provides services to terminally ill patients who have made the difficult decision to stop further "curative" treatment. Thus, hospice care isn't about *life* extension, but *quality* extension. Hospice addresses all end-stage disease aspects, including physical symptoms, psychological and social distress, and spiritual/emotional pain. Additional information about hospice care can be found at the National Hospice Foundation website at http://www.nationalhospicefoundation.org.

Eldercare   At its core, cancer is a disease of aging (80 percent of cancer cases occur in people age 50 and over). As such, eldercare—an umbrella term referring to the mix of community, social, financial, and medical services for people age 65 and over—helps millions meet the challenges of living with cancer. Eldercare services include, but aren't limited to, personal care, home health care, financial and estate planning, counseling, and transportation. An eldercare worker—typically a social worker or allied healthcare professional—might help a client review and receive health insurance coverage, or find a good estate attorney. Some eldercare agencies offer their services free of charge.

Meals on Wheels   Meals on Wheels delivers prepared meals if you want to stay at home during treatment but are unable to cook or don't have the financial resources to have someone do it for you. Many communities provide this service free for anyone 60 or older, regardless of income. Some even deliver to younger adults in need and homebound. Service fees vary and are available both long and short term.[7] See http://www.mealsonwheelsamerica.org for more information.

Adult Day Care   Adult day care (ADC) centers are places where people (usually older adults, but sometimes temporarily or permanently disabled people as young as 18) stay during the day so they are not alone in their homes. Supervision, help with daily living needs, personal grooming care, activities, and companionship are provided. Patients return home at night. Financial assistance is available for qualified individuals. Some of the services ADC centers provide may also include the following:

- Therapeutic and recreational activities (exercise, crafts, music, etc.)
- Medical care
- Counseling
- Education
- Supervision
- Meals
- Caregiver support groups or referral to other programs
- Transportation

For more information, call Eldercare Locator at 800-677-1116, or visit http://www.eldercare.gov/eldercare.NET/Public/index.aspx.

Assisted Living Facilities Assisted living facilities are options favored by older adults who value their independence but who also need help with daily living tasks. Across the country, millions of people call assisted living facilities home. Facilities and costs vary widely, but most offer some or all of the following services:

- Housing
- Meals
- 24-hour emergency monitoring
- Supervision and dispensing of medications
- Peer group support and socialization
- Assistance with bathing, dressing, grooming, eating, and/or transportation

Pulling It All Together

I can't stress it enough: Knowledge is power. Becoming a lung cancer expert puts you firmly in the driver's seat—the best position to find optimal care. Quality medical care is your right. And it starts with choosing a great cancer care team, then a quality treatment facility that will best meet your needs.

Step V

Remove Toxic Substances
from Your Life

CHAPTER 8

Stop Smoking Now!

Takeaways

- Although fewer than 20 percent of adult Americans smoke, cigarette smoking is a leading cause of disability and death in the United States and abroad.
- Lung cancer, chronic bronchitis, and emphysema incidence would drop more than 50 percent if people would simply stop smoking.
- A smoker is at 14 times greater risk of dying from cancer of the lung, throat, or mouth than a nonsmoker.
- According to the Centers for Disease Control and Prevention (CDC), 126 million nonsmoking Americans are at risk for tobacco-related diseases including lung cancer by exposure to secondhand smoke. Nonsmokers, especially the children and elderly, are at risk by exposure to "third-hand smoke," remnants from smoking that remain even if a smoker has left the area, by attaching to clothing, carpets, drapes, and other materials. Those "third-hand" remnants can enter a person's body through the skin, mouth, and respiratory system.
- Doctors should ask people about tobacco use at every office visit and provide counseling about quitting. Smokers should know how their habit interferes with potential treatment.
- Quitting is not easy. Many try, but only a few succeed. Quitting is an "it takes a village" mission. Doctors, families, spouses, friends, and even employers can be part of your village. Enlist their help.
- Parents still have the biggest impact on a child's decision to smoke. The best way to prevent your child from smoking is to stop smoking yourself, or not start in the first place.

- You've heard it before, but I will say it again: Quitting smoking lowers your risk of lung cancer greatly.

Introduction

Smoking kills.

It's no great revelation. Where do I even begin? Tobacco smoke contains carbon monoxide, the same gas found in automobile exhaust. Carbon monoxide is lethal, attaching to the body's red blood cells, depriving the heart and the rest of the body of oxygen. Other tobacco smoke compounds cause blood platelets to become sticky, increasing the likelihood of blood clots.[1]

Should I continue? Smoking increases the likelihood of complications from lung cancer treatments, specifically surgery, radiation therapy, and chemotherapy. Pneumonia, for example, is more common in smokers following surgery. Smokers cough up more mucus after surgery, spend more time on a ventilator, and have longer hospital stays. Smoking may intensify therapy-related fatigue and chemotherapy-related nausea, and may contribute to a decrease in appetite.

A single cigarette contains an estimated 600 ingredients. A burning cigarette releases 7,000 chemicals, the majority of which are toxic. In the United States, the mortality rate for smokers is three times that of people who never smoked, making it one of the leading causes of preventable death.[2]

Tobacco in any form kills. Cigarettes, marijuana, cigar, hookah, peace pipe, e-cigarettes—there's no safe way to smoke, period. Replacing your cigarette with a cigar, pipe, or even hookah won't help you avoid tobacco-associated health risk. Cigars have a higher level of carcinogens, toxins, and tar than cigarettes, reports the National Cancer Institute (NCI). Hookah smoke has many toxic compounds and exposes smokers to more carbon monoxide than cigarettes. Hookahs also produce more secondhand smoke.[3]

Cigarette smoking is the single greatest risk factor for lung cancer. Nothing else, including asbestos, comes close. Eighty-five percent of newly diagnosed lung cancer patients smoked for at least a decade before diagnosis. Why did you willingly do something so foolish? Did smoking help you relieve stress or anxiety? Did you want to look cool in front of your friends? Maybe you read somewhere that smoking is an effective appetite suppressant.

Whatever your reason for smoking, you also know it's damned hard to quit. It is an addiction. In fact, many lung cancer patients continue to smoke after diagnosis. In this way, they're no different than drug addicts (and nicotine *is* a hardcore drug). Withdrawal from nicotine causes nausea, headaches, psychological disorder, and a host of other potential symptoms. It *is* an addiction. You should quit—now. It's never too late to quit; there are literally 100 great reasons to go cold turkey and not a single good reason to keep smoking.

Nicotine's Deadly Reach

When it comes to the ingredients in tobacco, nicotine deservedly garners all the popcorn headlines. It takes just seconds for nicotine to reach your brain. Nicotine is a central nervous system stimulant, meaning you may even feel temporarily energized after using it. Once the effect subsides, however, you may crash and start craving it more and more. Nicotine, of course, is also habit forming. The more you use, the more you crave.

Smoking damages the entire cardiovascular system. Nicotine constricts blood vessels, restricting blood flow and causing peripheral artery disease. Smoking also lowers good cholesterol levels and raises blood pressure, which can result in stretching of the arteries and a buildup of LDL ("bad") cholesterol, leading to atherosclerosis. Smoking raises the risk of forming blood clots and seriously increases the risk of stroke.

Tobacco causes gum inflammation (gingivitis) or serious infection (periodontitis) problems, that may lead to tooth decay, tooth loss, and bad breath. Smoking, predictably, creates fertile ground for many forms of cancer, including lung, mouth, throat, laryngeal, and esophageal cancers. In addition, kidney and pancreatic cancers are more common among smokers than nonsmokers. Smoking puts you at greater risk for developing Type 2 diabetes. Even cigar smokers who don't inhale are at higher risk for mouth cancer.

If that's not enough to convince you to stop, consider how it damages the way you look and smell. The substances in tobacco smoke actually alter the skin's structure, increasing the likelihood of discoloration, wrinkles, and premature aging. Smoking stains teeth and fingertips yellow and brown. And the tobacco smell stays in your hair, as well as clothes.

If all of that is not enough, consider what it does to your sex life and sex organs. Smoking causes blood vessels to constrict, restricting blood flow to the penis and reducing the ability to get and maintain erections. It creates an obstacle to achieving orgasm for both men and women. Smokers of either gender are also at higher risk for infertility. Smoking can trigger early menopause and cervical cancer in women; and female smokers experience more pregnancy-related complications, including miscarriage, problems with the placenta, and premature delivery.[4]

Newborns of pregnant mothers exposed to secondhand smoke are more likely to have low weight, birth defects, and sudden infant death syndrome (SIDS). Newborns who breathe in secondhand smoke are more prone to ear and respiratory infections and asthma attacks.[5] Later in life, the children of smokers are at higher risk for respiratory disorders including asthma, wheezing and coughing, pneumonia, and bronchitis. They are also more prone to ear infections.

Smoking wreaks havoc on our eyes and increases the risk of age-related macular degeneration, cataracts, and vision loss.[6] It kills our sense of taste and smell, making food much less enjoyable. Physical withdrawal impairs cognitive functioning, leading us to feel anxious, irritated, and depressed. Withdrawal causes headaches and sleep problems.

Perhaps no organ takes a bigger hit from smoking than the lungs. Inhaling smoke—remember the earlier list of chemicals and toxins in cigarette and cigar smoke—damages the lungs, which eventually lose their ability to filter out the toxins, so some are trapped there. Best case, smokers start to experience more respiratory problems: repeated colds, bouts of flu, and infections. Worst case, they develop cancer.

Cigarette smoking is the major cause of emphysema, a condition that destroys your lungs' airways, and chronic bronchitis, another form of chronic obstructive pulmonary disease (COPD) where lung linings become inflamed.

News and the Real Scoop on Secondhand Smoke

The news is just in—seemingly good news, but don't let it give you a false sense of security. Although previous associations between health damage and secondhand smoke exposure have been widespread, one large study, which followed 76,000 women for more than a decade, found the usual link between smoking and cancer but concluded there was no "statistically significant" link between lung cancer and exposure to passive (secondhand) smoke. The study, published in the prestigious *Journal of the National Cancer Institute,* found only "borderline statistical significance" for the link between passive smoke and women who developed lung cancer after living with a smoker for 30 years or more.[7]

In other news, secondhand smoke exposure has declined by 50 percent since 2000, according to a report from the CDC. While an estimated 53 percent of nonsmokers tested positive for a nicotine marker in their blood in 2000, signaling exposure to secondhand smoke, only 25 percent of the nonsmokers tested positive for a nicotine marker in 2012. The trend, say CDC officials, can be traced to state and municipal smoking bans in bars, restaurants, and offices, and the fact that fewer Americans now smoke inside their homes.[8]

So should we stop worrying about the adverse effects of secondhand smoke? Have the much-ballyhooed effects of passive smoking all been much ado about nothing? Hardly! I laugh when researchers use terms like "borderline statistical significance." Either something is significant or it's not. For one thing, the study doesn't touch on many ill effects of breathing secondhand smoke, including asthma, cardiopulmonary disease (diseases that affect the heart and lungs) such as hypertension and COPD, and stroke. Really, the study, and accompanying headline, is misleading because it merely confirms what many of us already know: Low levels of passive exposure to secondhand smoke don't significantly increase the risk of lung cancer, but they can trigger a host of other problems, such as asthma and heart disease. The CDC estimates secondhand smoke is responsible for 46,000 preventable heart disease deaths and 3,400 preventable cancer deaths annually.

Although fewer people are exposed to secondhand smoke, a substantial share of nonsmokers—25 percent—are still exposed to secondhand smoke, which is why experts estimate that secondhand exposure causes 41,000 lung cancer deaths and heart disease and 400 SIDS deaths annually. Tobacco use in the single greatest cause of preventable death in the United States, killing on average nearly half a million people each year.

Secondhand smoke exposure hits minorities, the poor, and children the hardest. Nearly 50 percent of black nonsmokers were exposed to secondhand smoke in 2012, compared to approximately 20 percent of whites. Predictably, exposure is far higher, nearly twice as common, among poor people who don't smoke than it was among their counterparts with higher incomes. Sadly, children aged 3 to 11 were the age group most often exposed to secondhand smoke. Among those children, 40 percent of white children, 30 percent of Hispanic chiidren, and a whopping 70 percent of black children had been exposed.

Similarly, other studies found that black nonsmoking adults had higher exposure to secondary smoke, as determined by blood tests for cotinine, a "biomaker" for tobacco smoke exposure. Researchers leading these studies said blacks were more often exposed to smoke in their workplaces and that there is some evidence that cotinine stays in their systems longer than in people of other races.

What Is Third-Hand Smoke, and Is It Really Hazardous to Your Health?

It took decades for the public to wake up to the dangers associated with secondhand smoke. Now, another cigarette-related phenomenon is raising concern: third-hand smoke. Before you start laughing, know this: it's real, and it's ubiquitous.

Have you ever taken a whiff of a smoker's hair? Did you ever enter a room and wondered why it smelled like a dirty ashtray when there wasn't a cigarette butt in sight? This is third-hand smoke.

Third-hand smoke is the fallout from smoking, airborne elements that are toxic and build up over time. It's the stuff that lingers long after secondhand smoke has disappeared to the eye. It's in the smell, grunge, and yellowing on the environment where a smoker spends time. It's more noticeable in smaller space, such as a car. But third-hand smoke settles on and seeps into carpet and porous surfaces such as paneling or drywall, in addition to lingering on hair, skin, clothes, and fingernails. Yes, even smokers themselves emit deadly toxin, typically from their hair and clothing. So even if parents go outside to smoke, then enter the home to hold their son or daughter, they are exposing their innocent children to third-hand smoke.

Research has not been done to determine just how long toxins from third-hand smoke stay in the home, automobile, and other environments. However, we do know that the compounds in third-hand smoke are lethal to human health. Lead, for example, can lead to significant cognitive delays in children by damaging the frontal lobes of the brain, and cyanide is a compound that interferes with the release of oxygen to tissues. Like carbon monoxide, cyanide binds to hemoglobin, meaning it competes with oxygen for binding sites. Of greatest concern is the effect of third-hand smoke on the most vulnerable, including babies, toddlers, children, the sick, and the elderly. Babies crawl on carpets, sleep on fabric couches, and teeth on household and other porous objects, all of which may be invisibly dirtied with third-hand smoke toxins. The sick and elderly, both with compromised immune systems, spend a lot of time indoors and are especially at risk in places exposed to third-hand smoke.

Although any number of environmental toxins can contribute to lung cancer, cigarette smoke is far more lethal than toxins found in automobile exhaust and asbestos. One of these toxins, a tobacco-specific nitrosamine known as NNA, damages DNA, potentially causing cancer.[9]

The bottom line is that there's no such thing as a risk-free level of tobacco exposure.

Genetics of Tobacco Use and Dependence

Although many factors influence tobacco experimentation and the downward spiral to regular smoking, the risk of addiction appears to be significantly influenced by physiological factors that have an underlying genetic basis.

From twin studies, we know that smoking heritability ranges from 50 to 80 percent, placing it squarely in the same category as alcoholism. The genetic factors that influence initiation and dependence most certainly overlap, but there's compelling evidence that genes may act in each stage of tobacco use as well.

To date, large-scale studies have identified a limited number of the genes underlying addiction risk. Like the recent discovery of a genetic risk for obesity, it appears that multiple genes underlie smoking heritability, each having a small but cumulative effect on addiction risk. Studies of specific "candidate" (individual) genes have produced inconsistent findings, probably because it's virtually impossible to analyze a behavior like smoking where there's a complex interplay of genes and environment.

Genes might affect addiction susceptibility by upping the number and sensitivity of nicotine receptors, increasing the speed and efficiency of nicotine metabolism, and the physiological and behavioral responses to nicotine, which I discuss in greater detail later in this chapter. An inherited variation within the human *CYP2A6* gene, which influences the rate at which the body metabolizes nicotine, may affect tobacco consumption.[10]

Better aids to stop smoking may be developed with more research on the genetics of addiction, but pharmacological approaches still may not be effective against one singularly strong psychological element: environment. It is estimated as much as 50 percent of the risk of addiction is due to environmental factors. So government tobacco control policies to discourage all people from smoking still remain key to any antismoking effort.

A New Zealand study aimed to determine whether people with high genetic risk for tobacco addiction became addicted more easily as teenagers and whether that had a bearing on the success or failure of any later attempt to quit. The study followed 1,000 people from birth to age 38. Those who tried smoking as teenagers were more likely to become daily smokers and heavy (a pack a day or more) smokers. Those with a high-risk genetic factor smoked more and were less likely to quit. By age 38, they had smoked longer, were more likely addicted, and more likely to fail at attempts to quit.

In 2013, Duke University researchers, who also participated in the New Zealand study, scanned the entire genomes of tens of thousands of smokers.[11] What they saw overall among the heavy smokers were variations in genes that control how nicotine is metabolized and how the brain responds to nicotine. This allowed researchers to develop a "genetic risk scoring system," although we do not yet know, as of this writing, how the variations seen affect gene function.

In the New Zealand study, genetic risk was clearly tied to tobacco addiction. Early teenagers who had the high-risk genetic profile and tried cigarettes were 24 percent more likely to smoke daily by age 15, and within three years of that become pack-a-day smokers. As adults, people with genetics making them high risk for tobacco addiction were more often addicted and more likely to fail when trying to quit. By age 38, study participants with high-risk genetic profiles had smoked about 7,300 more cigarettes (equivalent of one "pack-year") than the average smoker.[12]

The researchers concluded that not becoming a regular, heavy smoker as a teen appeared to confer a sort of immunity to genetic risk for adult smoking problems. The takeaway—not just for teens, but also their parents—is that any genetic risk is limited to people who take up the habit during their teen years. From a medical perspective, the results suggest to me that nicotine exposure may have a special effect on the adolescent brain, especially as it relates to these gene variants, and may explain why the teen years are a period of highest risk of nicotine addiction.

How this genetic risk affects brain functions, which subsequently affect reactions to nicotine, is still unknown. In the interim, all we can do is preach the antismoking message and enact policies that make it harder for teenagers to get hold of cigarettes and become regular smokers as adults.

Addiction Anatomy 101: Why It's So Hard to Quit Smoking

For Jimmy, a former Super Bowl champion NFL lineman, it began with a single drag. From there, it progressed to half a pack. Before long, Jimmy was smoking up to two packs of cigarettes a day—while he was still playing! Jimmy smoked to deal with the stress, expectation, and uncertainty of life as a world-class athlete. After retiring, Jimmy continued smoking. In fact, he increased his daily intake to three packs a day, in part to deal with the reality of no longer doing something he loved and bringing home a regular paycheck. Recently, a mass was discovered on Jimmy's right lung during a pre-op chest X-ray before hernia surgery.

A month later, Jimmy was in my office for a consult after receiving a diagnosis of stage I adenocarcinoma, a type of non-small cell lung cancer (NSCLC). Fortunately for Jimmy, the cancer was still confined to his right lung and, according to his PET scan, hadn't spread to any surrounding lymph nodes.

The question I ask all new patients over age 55 isn't if they smoke, but when did they start. I know that a majority of my patients smoked at some point in their lives. To the baby boom generation, a pack of smokes is today's equivalent of the Smartphone: everyone had one. For many smokers, a lung cancer diagnosis is more than enough motivation to quit cold turkey. Yet, a substantial minority still smoke after their diagnosis. Jimmy was one of those patients.

Indeed, a study in the journal *Cancer* found more than one-third of cancer patients still smoked at the time of diagnosis, and even five months after diagnosis, nearly 15 percent of lung cancer patients still smoked. Most quit after diagnosis, which happened with Jimmy after we sat down for a very honest talk about what would happen if he didn't quit immediately.[13]

The thing about smoking is that the desire to quit, no matter how strong, is not always enough for them to succeed in beating the addiction. There are several factors that make quitting a challenge for even the most determined people.

For many people, like Jimmy, the problem starts with the first drag. In just a few seconds, cigarette smoke sends nicotine to the brain. Brain cells react by releasing pleasure center chemicals including dopamine. The nicotine grabs hold of receptors on brain cells, releasing a wave of dopamine and other pleasurable chemicals.

In response, brain cells sprout new nicotine receptors (nicotinic acetylcholine receptors, or nAChRs). The more you're exposed cigarette smoke, the more your brain produces new receptors. The more dopamine produced, the more a smoker, consciously or not, wants that pleasurable feeling, so he or she smokes more and becomes a pack-a-day, or worse, two-pack-a-day smoker. This is why it's so damn hard to quit smoking. It's not unlike the brain events for other drug addicts—from cocaine fiends to heroin junkies.

When you stop smoking, your dopamine supply drops, which leads to withdrawal. The fate of the brain's nicotine receptors once the nicotine supply runs dry is still unknown. Although it makes sense that the receptors would just die off, one study showed that common withdrawal symptoms including depression and tension persisting for more than month after the last puff. Research is under way to hopefully identify "targeted" drugs that could be used to temporarily stimulate the receptors in order to "wean" tobacco quitters from the pleasurable biochemicals so that they can resist the urge to light up.

Still, solving the dopamine craving doesn't make quitting easy. Smoking also releases other "feel-good" molecules in the brain, including endogenous opioids, which raise positive emotions while reducing negative ones. Moreover, dopamine might be why people get addicted to cigarettes, but blocking its rewarding effects isn't necessarily how a person gets better. There are lasting changes that occur in the brain after addiction. And addiction, like any chronic illness, has a strong behavioral component that can't be fixed with a pill. Unlike heroin or other illicit drugs, cigarettes are easy to come by, and even in the age of public smoking bans, you can still light up legally in your car or home.

Socioeconomic variables factor in as well. Lung cancer patients who continue smoking following diagnosis are most often single, uninsured, sicker, more depressed, and heavier smokers. A study in the journal *Cancer* found that 14 percent of lung cancer patients still smoked months after diagnosis and were less likely to have undergone surgery to treat their cancer.[14] This may be because many surgeons insist patients stop smoking before surgery, which is exactly what I did with Jimmy. I explained to him that quitting would speed his recovery and wound healing and decrease postoperative complications such as pneumonia. With major surgery, you need all the help you can get. I also insisted that Jimmy get a blood test to detect carbon monoxide levels. I took action to impress on Jimmy how serious I was about his quitting before surgery. He knew I meant business when I said I wouldn't operate on him if he didn't quit.

Patients with advanced-stage lung cancer also had higher rates of smoking after diagnosis, reflecting a belief that quitting wouldn't positively affect their chances of survival. When it comes to quitting smoking, late-stage lung cancer patients present an interesting challenge. As a doctor, I want to point out the detrimental effects of continuing the habit that brought them into my office in the first place. But as a friend, I don't want to take away something that brings pleasure. However, I don't often see myself in the position of having to convince people to quit, regardless of the stage of their disease. In fact, after a decade as a practicing thoracic surgeon, I can count on one hand the number of patients who kept smoking after our initial consult.

Clearly, it's possible to quit, but it's by no means an easy road.

The Road Forward: Quitting for Good

Lung cancer treatment has come a long way in the last decade. Still, even the most up-to-date treatments inevitably damage normal lung tissue. This is often true with surgery, when some surrounding lung tissue must be excised to extract all of the cancer. Radiation therapy, on the other hand, which can also damage normal cells, leading to side effects, has evolved enough where it can sometimes be targeted in patients where the cancer has spread to only a few sites (these treatments minimize the amount of normal lung tissue affected by the radiation beams). More recently, new "targeted" drugs (discussed in

Chapter 5), including angiogenesis inhibitors and anti-EGFR drugs, among others, have been developed to counter and even reverse the growth of lung cancer cells.[15]

As with all lung cancer treatments, there are side effects, some of which can be severe. Doesn't it make sense then to quit smoking and conserve as much lung functioning as possible? Of course it does. *This is why smoking cessation is the most important part of any lung cancer treatment program!* Quitting smoking increases the likelihood of a positive response to treatment. Quitting smoking can prevent or lessen the severity of other medical problems. Smoking, as an example, increases the formation of dangerous blood clots. Clots forming in blood vessels that carry oxygen to the heart can lead to a heart attack; clots forming in blood vessels in the brain may lead to a stroke.

Even if you've been smoking for years, quitting smoking today can slow further loss of lung function. Quitting smoking may also help prevent the development secondary lung cancer (the precancerous changes that eventually turned into a cancerous tumor in one area may also be present in other parts of the lungs). Research has shown that even patients with a successfully treated early-stage lung cancer have a 2 to 3 percent chance per year of developing secondary lung cancer.[16]

Going Cold Turkey: Your Plan to Quit

Since no two people are alike, find a method that works best for you. Some people simply make the decision to quit and never touch tobacco again. However, for most smokers, quitting is hard and requires some major planning. Smoking cessation experts recommend picking a "quit date." It's a matter of choice whether you decide to gradually taper off until your quit date or whether you plan to smoke until that day before going cold turkey.

Many smokers experience their first "a-ha" quit moment after surgery or other lung cancer treatment. This is a great time to quit because you're in a supportive environment with doctors, nurses, and others to answer your questions and keep you on the straight and narrow. You can have instant access to smoking cessation drugs, and I can assure you no one will light up at the hospital. No access, fewer triggers, more support, and a whole lot of down time make the hospital an ideal place to pause and reflect on your smoking triggers—specific events, situations, and even people that send you running for tobacco.

Identify Your Triggers

Smoking is like overeating. And just like overeating, you'll see that smokers have predictable patterns. When, where, and at what time do you light up? Addictive behavior is all about habit patterns. Look at your own life and you'll see a distinctive pattern to your smoking. Do you reach for a pack after a heavy meal, while driving, or talking on the phone? Or do you reach for cigarettes along with the first cup of morning coffee? Do smoke breaks give you time to talk to friends at work? Once you've identified some of your smoking triggers, you can come up with strategies for dealing with them when they surface in your daily life. Decide how you will handle them effectively. Remember, the desire or urge to light up lasts only three to five minutes. Experts recommend coming up with a list of things to do other than smoking when cravings hit. Try blocking-behaviors such as taking a walk, drinking water, trying some controlled breathing exercises (recommended elsewhere in this book), or practicing stress management. Sucking on hard candy or "puffing" on a straw can keep your hands busy and mind occupied. And don't be surprised if you crave cigarettes long after the pangs of withdrawal vanish. Smoking is a complex behavior that involves more than simply removing nicotine from your life.

Smoking Cessation Programs

Smoking cessation programs can be of enormous benefit when you're trying to quit. If you've been diagnosed with lung cancer, you're already dealing with a boatload of stuff, and you may appreciate help from a smoking cessation program. The best programs view tobacco addiction as a chronic disease and recommend strategies to help people quit smoking. These strategies include education, emotional support, medications, and relapse prevention. Choose a program that emphasizes behavioral change, since at the heart of every chronic illness is a behavioral component. Programs offer both individual counseling and support groups.

Drug Therapy

Drug therapy can be an important component of a smoking cessation program. Nicotine replacement drugs and other medications have proved effective in helping smokers quit. Drug therapy plays an important role in smoking cessation. Two types of drugs are used to help people quit smoking: nicotine replacements and non-nicotine-containing prescription medications. Both are designed to ease symptoms of withdrawal such as irritability, frustration, anger, anxiety, poor concentration, restlessness, and depression.[17]

Nicotine Gum   Nicotine polacrilex is an over-the-counter nicotine gum. Basic instructions call for chewing the gum slowly until you feel a mild tingling, which is the nicotine being released. Then place the gum between your cheek and gums for several minutes before chewing it again. This technique provides for gradual absorption of the nicotine and should continue for 30 minutes per piece of gum. Many of my patients find that 10 to 15 pieces of gum per day are needed to quit smoking. Nicotine lozenges that dissolve in your mouth are also available.[18]

Nicotine Patches   One of the most popular smoking cessation aids, the nicotine patch provides a steady controlled dose of nicotine throughout the day. Nicotine patches, obtained by a prescription, resemble adhesive bandages. Each contains a layer of nicotine that's absorbed though the skin before entering your bloodstream. The patches should be placed on a comfortable, hairless site on the skin. Don't exceed the recommended dosage unless otherwise advised by your physician. However, your doctor may prescribe a higher dosage (wearing more than one patch at a time) if you are a heavy smoker. Side effects may include mild skin irritation. Many smokers worry about the patch's having an addictive component, but believe me, patches have much lower levels of nicotine than cigarettes. So, don't be afraid of nicotine patches, especially if they help you quit smoking.[19]

Nicotine Nasal Spray   Nicotine nasal spray, sold under the brand-name Nicotrol NS, works by delivering nicotine to your body via the nostrils. Most people use about 15 doses per day, decreasing the number over time. This spray can be used successfully up to twelve weeks. It works especially well for heavy smokers.[20]

Nicotine Inhaler   A nicotine inhaler resembles a cigarette and contains a small capsule filled with nicotine-treated cotton. Puffing on the device delivers vaporized nicotine to the linings of the mouth and upper throat where it is absorbed. It may be the best choice for anyone who needs the ritual or "feel" of smoking. Unlike a nicotine patch, which delivers a constant level of nicotine, nicotine inhalers produce a more rapid increase in nicotine levels in the blood, followed by a decrease in nicotine levels—more like an actual cigarette. Possible side effects include mild throat irritation, runny nose, watering eyes, sneezing, coughing, and a hot, peppery feeling in the nose or the back of the throat.

Chantix   Chantix is the brand-name for the non–nicotine drug varenicline. It works by blocking the pleasurable effects of nicotine. Chantix comes in pill form and is usually taken once or twice a day to start. The drug needs time to build up in your body, so it's recommended that you begin taking Chantix a week before you give up smoking completely. You may smoke during the first week, but you should go cold turkey on the eighth day of treatment. The most common side effects of Chantix are nausea, insomnia, constipation, gas, and vomiting. People taking Chantix may need to be observed for any subsequent psychological problems because there have been reports of depression and suicidal thoughts among a small segment of Chantix users.[21]

Zyban   The prescription drug Zyban is the brand-name for the drug bupropion, the first medication approved by the Food and Drug Administration (FDA) for smoking cessation. It comes in pill form and does not contain nicotine. The drug reduces withdrawal symptoms by stimulating the release of the same brain chemicals released in response to nicotine. These chemicals improve alertness, concentration, and memory. Zyban also stimulates the brain's pleasure centers—the ventral tegmental area (VTA) and the nucleus accumbens, to name a few—mimicking other nicotine side effects. Patients are usually instructed to continue smoking for two weeks after starting Zyban, as it enables the drug to build up in the body before you quit. Zyban isn't without risks, however. Frequently seen side effects include anxiety, changes in appetite, constipation, diarrhea, dizziness, drowsiness, dry mouth, headache, increased sweating, nausea, nervousness, stomach pain, stuffy nose, trouble sleeping, vomiting, and weight changes.[22]

When You Finally Decide to Quit

It may seem hokey, but set a definite "quit date." The human mind responds well to boundaries. On that day, remove all forms of temptation from your home because this is the place you're most likely to smoke, especially given the public restriction and social stigma surrounding smoking. Dispose of all tobacco, lighters, and ashtrays. Tell someone else about your plan—someone willing to hold you accountable, like a spouse or close friend. Ask your doctor about medications that can help treat nicotine withdrawal. Be prepared to handle cravings and to feel discomfort for the first week or two. Expect to be less productive, so plan a lighter workload. Avoid situations that trigger smoking. Have low-calorie snacks available. Quit for one day at a time. Reward yourself for your success. If you slip, which is certainly possible, don't get discouraged. Start back on your plan.

It takes persistence and dedication to give up smoking. Experts say that most people make numerous serious attempts before actually quitting for good (five years and seven attempts, according to a well-publicized British study).[23]

If you do have a slip, try to understand what caused you to want to smoke. Plan to handle that situation differently next time. Then, set another quit date and try again. Once you have quit, reward yourself. Remember, too, that you'll need to stay vigilant—remaining a nonsmoker requires effort. It may be a while before you stop thinking about having a cigarette.

Step VI
Acceptance

CHAPTER 9

Your Life with Lung Cancer

Takeaways

- There are a number of ways to cope with problems, some healthy, others not.
- How do you deal with a lung cancer diagnosis? To start, understand and admit your feelings about living with lung cancer. It's the first step to ensuring that you receive the best possible treatment.
- Don't spurn the affections or interests of those who care about you. A cancer diagnosis has a ripple effect.
- Don't lose hope. It's an essential part of living with lung cancer, regardless of your prognosis.

Introduction

Let's put all our cards on the table: A diagnosis of lung cancer sucks, just as I said earlier in the book. "A double shot to the head and the stomach" is how one patient ever so elegantly described it. You'll probably feel powerful emotions surface, from shock to fear, denial to anger, and everything in between. Don't hang your head in shame, however. You've just been told you have a life-threatening illness. You're not normal if you're not at your wit's end after learning this news.

A lung cancer diagnosis ranks up there with swimming with man-eating sharks and playing Russian roulette. Dealing with the disease's many challenges is no day at beach. I tell my patients that a lung cancer diagnosis falls in the "unnecessary stress" category. Who the hell needs this? I know the old adage about growing and learning from our experiences, but there are other ways to learn life lessons than having cancer.

Patients ask me about the appropriate way to handle a lung cancer diagnosis. The question is impossible to answer as though there's a school of etiquette for dealing with life-threatening illnesses. "Pull yourself together," I remember one family member telling another. Easy for him to say; he wasn't the one contemplating surgery, recovery, and months of painful and debilitating chemo and radiation. What if the shoe were on the other foot? Stress is part of the deal. How we react to it is the true definition of self.

There's no right or wrong way to cope with a lung cancer diagnosis. In fact, here's a bit of advice: Cope with it in your way, whatever that may be. I'm not here to lecture you or tell you how to deal. I treat patients, but I don't have lung cancer. You live with this disease. I just want to provide you with enough information to help you cope in your way. Successful coping strategies don't match some arbitrary criteria. But all great coping strategies do have one thing in common: They contribute to well-being.

Following a diagnosis, your plate will fill quickly. First of all, you're going to have to come to terms with the news. Denial won't do you much good, I'm afraid. Unless you've been squatting in a remote mountain cave for the better part of 20 years, you're going to have to spill the beans to someone at some point.

While you're trying to deal with this bewildering array of pitches, life will throw you something entirely unexpected before you're remotely ready to step into the batter's box. You're entering a brave new medical world. If you're not overwhelmed, at least initially, there just might be something wrong with you. New words, alien procedures, treatment decisions, financial pressures, and family concerns—these are just a handful of the many challenges you'll face. The first few weeks can throw you for a loop if you're not prepared. Beyond a doctor announcing, "you're cured," my goal is to help you discover a way to live and thrive with lung cancer.

I have yet to meet a patient, even a hardened smoker, who wasn't shaken to the core after learning he or she has lung cancer. "Stunned," "bewildered," "numb"—common feelings after hearing the diagnosis. Numbness, a deeply encoded childhood coping strategy, is an alarming emotion nonetheless, especially for proactive people used to taking the bull by the horns when it comes dealing with the slings and arrows of life's misfortunes. Numbness is how we avoid coming apart at the seams. How was your thinking after hearing the news?

Disorganized, I bet, your mind filled with questions and concerns of what should be, what is, and what might be. "Why did this happen to me?" "How long have I got?" "Who will look after my family?" "Will the treatment work?" These are all common questions without easy, pat answers.

Grief is the universal human emotion. If you live on this planet, it's something you will experience many times. The psychiatrist Elisabeth Kübler-Ross first proposed the five stages of loss and mourning in her pioneering 1969 book, *On Death and Dying*. Lung cancer patients commonly experience these five stages. They are as follows:

- **Denial and Isolation**—These are feelings of shock and numbness. They're a denial of the new reality on the ground and a perfectly normal way of rationalizing overwhelming emotions. It's how even perfectly rational people deal with the first wave of grief upon learning that someone close to them has died or is terminally ill.
- **Anger**—After a certain amount of time, no one can continue to hide or deny reality. Once this happens, pain, which denial masked, emerges. Those who can't deal with the pain, and few can at this point, react in anger. This is target-less anger that can, and often is, directed at the universe, God, the people around you, your doctor, a complete stranger, or yourself. You may point the finger at your dying or deceased relative. You know this is crazy, right? But you resent the pain he's causing you. Of course, you feel guilty about being angry, which just makes you angrier. This is the second step's vicious cycle.
- **Bargaining**—This really falls into the "stinking thinking" category. You're burdened with unwarranted guilt, so you try to fix things. You need to regain control. You think of what you could've done differently. "If only I'd gotten a second opinion, things would be different." You may even enter into some weird, Faustian bargain. You're still looking for some protection from reality.
- **Depression**—The reality of the situation begins to set in; sadness, regret, and despair overwhelm you. You start worrying about everything. You need reassurance. Privately, you may also be preparing for the reality that is your new life after loss.
- **Acceptance**—This is an acknowledgment of your new life. It's a calmer place, and you may even feel more hopeful, motivated, and at peace. But this isn't a place that everyone gets to. It

involves letting go. We humans form attachments; we don't part easily with the things we cling to. Attachment leads to suffering of course, but what's the alternative? Someone can tell you how she or he thinks you should cope and move on, but that may not be your reality. No one can tell you how to feel. Dealing with loss and grief is a singular experience—ultimately you must travel this road alone. You can lean on others for support, but this is your journey. Allow yourself to grieve. Resisting or denying only prolongs the healing process.[1]

Fluctuating from one place to another during the acceptance process is common. At some point, you may even wonder if you're flirting with sanity. You're OK, and reacting in a perfectly acceptable way to a life-altering event. Human emotions color and enrich the experience of living. However, emotions that run high or boil over may cause us to momentarily lose our way.

Intense emotions need an outlet. Talking helps, a lot, and there are cancer patients who easily express their emotions. Others are more guarded. There's no right or wrong way. However, even the most emotionally stable person needs an outlet.

While it's important to share feelings, you might find your usual support people are rattled by your diagnosis. They're in shock. They may feel guilty. Trust me, they're experiencing the same sadness and fears as you. Under the circumstances, they may not be able to provide the support you need, at least not immediately. It's a lousy situation, but not at all uncommon.

Fortunately, there are a number of organizations available to help support you during your lung cancer journey. Some are limited to lung cancer patients; others include people with a wide range of cancers. Groups like Gilda's Club (on whose Board of Directors I serve) offer support to cancer patients and their families, providing an outlet for sharing concerns, information, and resources.

Coping Styles: How Do You Deal?

Anxiety and depression are a cancer patient's constant companions. Personality style, cultural upbringing, religious/spiritual beliefs, life circumstances, and outlook are among the many factors that influence how we cope. There is no all-purpose, "right" way to deal with cancer, only helpful and harmful coping skills. Anything that reduces anxiety and distress and helps you would fall into the "helpful" category.

We all cope differently. Cancer patients look for ways to regain control of a situation that appears out of control. Most newly diagnosed lung cancer patients don't know a CT scan from an X-ray. So information is key. Knowledge allays fear, anxiety, and feelings of helplessness. Good doctors diagnose and treat their patients. Great doctors, on the other hand, explain things and make their patients feel comfortable, even under the most trying circumstances. The best feeling any doctor—myself included—can have is having a patient leave with a clear blueprint of what lies ahead.

Some people find distracting themselves from the anxiety that comes from living with lung cancer helpful. It's a way of refocusing, or more precisely, redirecting their attention. "Distraction" carries a pejorative connotation, but it's also an effective way to reduce anxiety and stress. Pleasant diversions, like listening to music, reading, or taking a walk in the woods, are distractive coping mechanisms.

Most people tend to prefer one type of coping strategy but may enlist another when it best meets a need. Picture yourself in a traffic jam, as unpleasant as that may be. It's stressful and probably leaves you feeling irritated. Have you given any thought to an alternate route? What about getting off the nearest exit and grabbing a cup of coffee while you wait for the traffic to pass? These are effective coping strategies. Grabbing an MP3 player and zoning out to your favorite music would qualify as a distractive coping mechanism. These coping strategies can be used alone and together.

If you're like most cancer patients, you will probably find that, at some point, you'll fall back on a range of coping skills. You may also find it necessary to develop new coping strategies. Remember, there is no blueprint for dealing with cancer. You have to find the path that works for you.

Find a coping style that suits your temperament and needs. Some people are "all hands on deck." They're information junkies; the more they know, the better they feel. Others opt for a more laid-back approach, although people in this category are more the exception than the rule. They place decision-making authority in their doctor's hands, preferring to focus on the business of everyday living. There's no right or wrong way. You may opt for a middle ground. Whatever your coping style, share it with your doctor and other health care providers. It will help reduce the stress and anxiety associated with living with lung cancer.

Belief goes a long way here as well. Have faith in your ability to cope. It will help you function better. Belief is the first step to making it happen. Be confident that, even in the midst of the most trying circumstances, you will somehow pull through. You may not even know how you're going to go about doing this. However, you've probably faced a number of trying circumstances in your life. Cancer is no walk in the park, but it's not beyond your ability to deal with, either.

Obstacles to Coping

Don't Deny Your Feelings

In the last decade, the mind–body interaction and its effect on the course and progression of disease have drawn much interest. There are studies suggesting a link between how someone copes and his or her chances of surviving cancer. From my own experience working with patients, I'm convinced that attitude influences a patient's chance for surviving.[2]

Cancer patients who are told how they should feel or cope shoulder a great burden. I've heard doctors and other health care workers tell patients they need a "positive" attitude to survive cancer. Sure, that makes sense, but what if someone doesn't have the best attitude? What if he's understandably wary or fearful? What if she's overly burdened with guilt and shame?

We all know the benefits of adopting a positive outlook. However, the reality of living with lung cancer is that there will be many days when dread overwhelms all else. You will feel scared as often as you feel positive. Denying or suppressing your real feelings is far more detrimental to your health and happiness than facing them honestly or sharing them with others. Your feelings are your feelings. Some days you'll feel good; others days dread will hover over you like a ceaseless gray cloud. There really are no good or bad feelings. You can't be positive 24/7—cancer or not. You'll have bad days. You will feel angry, guilty, and confused. Just accept and live for each day. What other choice do you have?

Guilt and Blame

The smoking–lung cancer link has fueled the imagination of millions of lung cancer patients. They see their cancer as a self-inflicted wound. Since it's become clear that smoking is awful in every sense of the word, there's a fairly vocal and active segment of the population, both in and outside the public sector, willing to wave the antismoking flag. Still, there's an awful lot of latent resentment toward people who smoke or have smoked. Bad choices don't make you a bad person. "Blame" is an extra burden shouldered by lung cancer patients. It's a terrible, sad, traumatic, damn unfair situation having to fight cancer; no one deserves cancer! Take that to heart and keep it in your thoughts. It is a critical point. No one deserves cancer!

Judgmental feelings and finger-wagging about unhealthy lifestyle choices trigger much of the guilt and blame lung cancer patients experience. However, a majority of smokers start during their teens, a time when few people exercise the best judgment. And despite what you might hear from e-cigarette manufacturers, nicotine isn't a choice; it's a full-blown physical and psychological addiction.[3] The U.S. National Institute on Drug Abuse confirms the findings of a British report noting that 90 percent of people who try to quit smoking on their own (about 35 million Americans each year) relapse within one year, most going back to smoking within one week. Research has shown that nicotine is at least as addictive, or more addictive, than illegal drugs including cocaine and heroin (Blakeslee 1987). An advisory group of the British Royal College of Surgeons concluded most don't smoke because they choose to but because they are addicted. The U.S. National Institute on Drug Abuse also reported that, of the millions who quit each year without assistance, only 10 percent succeed in staying smoke-free for at least a year, and the vast majority don't last a full week.

Finger-pointing is ubiquitous among lung cancer patients. Self-blame is the noxious trap that cancer patients fall into. "If only I didn't smoke, this wouldn't have happened to me." This is stinking thinking. And it's wasted time. Self-blame blocks the path forward and keeps you from dealing with your diagnosis. Frequently, guilt triggers depression, making it all but impossible for patients to actively participate in their treatment. My advice: Stop blaming yourself, now. Who the hell wants to get lung cancer? Lung cancer isn't a form of divine retribution or karmic justice, even if you spent the majority of your life being a jerk. It's not your fault that you have lung cancer, even if you puffed away like a chimney for the better part of 30 years. I know plenty of two-pack-a-day smokers who, to this day, wash down their cigarettes with BLTs and beers and are still alive and kicking well into their 90s. On the other hand, I've treated people with advanced, aggressive lung cancer who never touched a cigarette. Life is seldom fair.

If you're feeling guilty or blaming yourself, work through these feelings. Consider talking to a therapist if you can't unburden yourself, or

seek out the guidance and wisdom of family, friends, and other supportive people. Self-blame is a major energy suck, and you'll need
every ounce of energy to help you adjust to living with lung cancer.
Whatever course you decide, let go of any guilt or blame you're experiencing. You've got bigger fish to fry.

When to Ask for Help

Depression hits us all. It's a normal response to a sad, disappointing,
unexpected, and/or stressful situation. "Reactive depression" is a way
of describing a perfectly normal response to a variety of adverse life
situations, including a diagnosis of a potentially life-threatening illness
like lung cancer. With the depression most people experience at—and
after—diagnosis, there is also anxiety, a routine feeling of unease (some
might call it "dis-ease"), worry, or even dread. Your heart may be racing, and you're having difficulty focusing. These are all normal reactions after a cancer diagnosis. But these normal, even healthy responses
can interfere with your life and health. The National Institute of Mental
Health lists the following common depression and anxiety symptoms.

Common Depression Symptoms

- Persistent sadness or anxiety
- An "empty" feeling
- Feelings of hopelessness or pessimism
- Feelings of guilt, worthlessness, or helplessness
- Loss of interest or pleasure in hobbies and activities that you
  once enjoyed, including sex
- Decreased energy, fatigue, or feeling slowed down
- Difficulty concentrating, remembering, or making decisions
- Insomnia or sleeping too much
- Appetite and/or weight loss, or overeating
- Persistent thoughts of death or suicide
- Restlessness or irritability
- Persistent headaches that are not attributable to another cause
  and do not respond to treatment[4]

Common Anxiety Symptoms

- Sweating
- Dizziness

- Racing heart or irregular heartbeat
- Shakiness
- Headaches
- Irritability/restlessness
- Sleeping problems
- Gastrointestinal distress, nausea, and/or diarrhea
- Difficulty concentrating
- Excessive watchfulness
- Being easily startled[5]

If these intense feelings are disrupting your life—affecting your ability to function—be sure to discuss the situation with your doctor or other health care provider. Counseling, medication, or another form of therapy may help. Don't ignore these symptoms. You're not losing your mind. You're not weak. You are coping with a shock. But anxiety and depression do need to be controlled if they're interfering with your quality of life.

The Hard Part: Breaking the Bad News

Sharing a cancer diagnosis with a spouse or partner is challenging. Sometimes it's hard to know where to begin. Learning a loved one has cancer is one of the most shocking, scary, and saddening events across most people's lifetimes. While you may want to remain silent about your cancer and spare loved ones that pain, it is usually not a good thing to do. If you were not in this situation, but your spouse, child, close friend, or other loved one was diagnosed with cancer, would you want to be kept in the dark? Wouldn't you want to be trusted with the news and given the option to support that person in whatever way you can? Generally, the sooner you tell people after diagnosis, the better. Many people find their partner or best friend becomes their main support across the lung cancer experience.

Keeping secrets isn't the best option. Let those who love you support you.

When I was a 19-year-old college sophomore, my father called to tell me that he was going on a business trip to Germany. I got a call a few days later that he'd just undergone heart surgery in New York City. I took the next flight out and drove into the city. When I saw him, I felt both relief and anger. I was angry because he didn't give me the chance to support him before a major operation. Every time he'd leave after that, I didn't know if he was going in for another medical procedure. I felt cut out of this important part of his life. I know he meant well and was trying to protect me, but our relationship took a hit. A little bit of trust was lost. The moral here is give your loved ones a chance to support you, no matter what you think is best.

How do you tell your partner or spouse you have lung cancer? It all depends on your relationship and how you cope, both as a couple and as individuals. Although the two of you may not have faced a cancer diagnosis, you've probably dealt with any number of challenging situations. Fall back on those experiences. What helped you get through challenging times before? Use them to guide you through the process of sharing your diagnosis.

Be aware that his or her feelings in response to the diagnosis will mirror many of yours, but will differ in some ways, too. Your partner may not know the best way to help you. People fumble and even lose their way because they don't know what to do. Your partner may want to try to pick up the slack, even taking over many of the things you normally do. Your partner or spouse may worry about money but is loath to broach the subject under the circumstances. The thought of even possibly having to live without you might bring more pain than they can cope with initially, but they might try to hide this fear to avoid causing you anguish or pain. The concern doesn't miraculously vanish, though. Few people go cold turkey on love. In time, you will open up and start talking about your feelings. Exploring painful and powerful emotions is healing.

Lung cancer will challenge both you and your spouse or partner. Personality style and coping skills affect the way you and your spouse or loved one cope with your diagnosis. Some partnerships are collaborative, where all decision making is done together. There are equally loving, but also fiercely independent people who divide their responsibilities. There's no right way to cope with your diagnosis. Find the way that works best for you and respects and honors your relationship.

Your Children

Parents want to protect their kids from distressing news, so they avoid sharing the cancer diagnosis with their children. Although your intentions may be honorable, keeping your diagnosis secret isn't in their—or your—best interests. My children hear everything. They know when Mommy and Daddy are trying to keep things private. They know more than we realize and worry if they think we're keeping something important from them. Avoiding difficult topics like a cancer diagnosis makes things worse in the long run. Your children, in particular, will start imagining worst-case scenarios.

Often, the bond among family members is strong enough that children will know when something is wrong. It doesn't matter how old or young they are, children sense when something is wrong. With young children, there's a fine line between honesty and giving them age-appropriate information. Younger kids will necessarily require simpler explanations. Regardless of age, be specific with your kids. Don't dance around the word "cancer" when talking about illness. Specificity reduces confusion and misunderstanding, especially if they happen to eavesdrop on a private conversation. If you have more than one child, don't be concerned if they start sharing information with their siblings. This helps them work things out in their own minds. Family members who deal best with a cancer diagnosis talk out the details, together. Honest and open communication allays confusion and ensures that misleading or inaccurate information doesn't make its way through your family.

Remind your children also that they're not to blame for your illness. Magical thinking is part of growing up, and youngsters may feel they are somehow responsible when bad things happen in their small world. Be clear with your children that they're not to blame for your illness. Repeat this message. They're trying to make sense of a situation that's not entirely clear to them.

Children learn by repetition, so they will ask the same questions again and again. Answer your children's questions consistently and honestly. Remind them that cancer isn't contagious. Be aware that older kids will pepper you with more detailed questions. If you don't have or know an answer, say so. Saying "I don't know" is OK. This is a good strategy, provided you do come back later with an answer to their question. Children are more aware and a hell of a lot smarter than we give them credit for. I was just six when my parents divorced. Separately, both reassured me that it wasn't my fault. They reminded me of this so often that I knew it wasn't my fault.

The $64 Million Question

"Are you going to die?"

If your child is old enough to understand the concept, he or she will almost certainly ask this question. This is a question no parent wants to answer. Young children, in particular, see parents as a safety net and fear losing them. They live in the moment, the present, not often thinking of the past or future—beyond what's for supper. So keep the answer in the present. Offer a realistic but honest assessment of your situation. Talk about all that's being done to treat your cancer. If they tell you they're scared, you might want to share that you're scared as well. If they see you crying or upset, tell them that crying is OK and perfectly normal.

The truth is, we're all living on borrowed time. As the best-selling author R. A. Salvatore so beautifully described it, "We are all dying, every moment that passes of every day. That is the inescapable truth of this existence." So when a child asks, it's OK to say, "We're all going to die some day. We just don't know when. But my doctors and I are doing everything we can to make sure I'm alive for a very long time."

Here's another thing to consider: Children are fairly resilient. They regularly surprise us with their coping skills and ability to adapt, even the face of adversity. Give your children a chance to help. Involve them in the process, but just be careful not to overwhelm them or give them more than they can handle. Sharing your cancer experience will help your kids as much as it benefits you.

Your Parents

"Parents shouldn't have to bury their children," a patient once told me. True, in theory, but real life doesn't always follow the script we write for ourselves. Most parents expect their children to outlive them, but this doesn't always happen. Losing a child is any parent's greatest fear. They're likely to experience the same range of powerful emotions that you and your spouse/partner felt after receiving a lung cancer diagnosis. Love, worry, and a heightened sense of responsibility overwhelm many parents, triggering feelings of guilt. "Is there something I could've done to prevent your cancer?"

Some parents infantilize their adult children when they get sick. If this is your parents' habit, tell them how this makes you feel. Your parents want to help, but don't know what to do or how to cope. So they fall back into old patterns that no longer work for you and your life. Take charge. Make your parents feel wanted and useful. They need this, and so do you. Give your parents a specific job. Those of you who are parents yourselves can relate to the fact that they want to do everything they can to help you recover. As a father, my children's happiness is paramount. I'd take the beating heart out of my chest if I knew it would spare them even a month's worth of pain and suffering. But also recognize this: They may need support of their own, especially to cope with irrational guilt about your situation. You may raise this issue with them and suggest finding friends, support groups, or a counselor to help.

How, When, and What to Tell Others

Another challenging aspect about having cancer is sharing the news with those outside your immediate family members. Brother and sisters, aunts and uncles, cousins, coworkers, and friends—you have to spill the beans at some point.

As with the members of your immediate family, you don't know how these people are going to react. Will they cry? Will they be numb or, worse, indifferent? A close friend or family member might jump in with both feet first, even offering to be your cancer point person. Others may not know how to cope. You even sense them pulling away, which has more to do with them or how they cope than with anything you might have done or said.

There are no easy answers. Sometimes it's best to see how someone else reacts. Do they seem interested in learning more about you and your condition? Do they seem willing or interested in helping? Would they rather talk about anything other than your diagnosis or condition?

Again, people cope with stress in different ways. Don't judge, no matter how painful it may be. Back off a bit. If someone cares about you, he or she will come around. If not, look elsewhere. There will be people willing to support you on your cancer journey. You'll find many people like this in your life.

If you have a job, don't wait to share your diagnosis with your boss or colleagues. You're going to need time off for treatment. Patients ask me all the time about approaching employers. I tell them: Cut to the chase. Approaching your boss early will foster trust and give you both peace of mind.

At first, your diagnosis will, of course, be a shock for people. But your loved ones will be glad you told them so they can help support you, and you will be better off with their help.

Epilogue

A Word or Two About Hope

Hope is a great power that can take many different forms. Hope comes from seeing the daily joys of life, life's meaning and purpose. What brings happiness and joy may be music to one person, the giggle of a baby, licks of a puppy, or even the beauty of a sunrise to another. It may be a friend's corny jokes, playing cards with a buddy, or just cuddling with a partner, for another. Things that inspire happiness and joy can change with our ages and stages and differ from person to person. We all have them, although sometimes we don't take the time to notice

What inspires hope in you? The answer depends on your values, beliefs, what gives your life meaning, and what makes you feel satisfied. And those answers can change with age and life phase. So think about it, what inspires hope in you?

During your cancer journey, your hopes may change. Doubt may sneak in, but there will always be reason to hope, no matter what the diagnosis or prognosis. Let your definition of hope be broad enough that you don't miss any chances for hope that are before you.

Hope is a great thing. It's not about holding onto unrealistic expectations or a belief in magic cures. Hope is what drives us to survive until we take our final bow. Don't despair if you're among the handful of patients who doesn't want to fight. You're not a failure. I can't tell you how many patients tell me out of earshot of their loved ones that they're tired of fighting. They're not throwing in the towel. Many simply want to live out the remainder of their lives in comfort.

A little handholding goes along way. My patients and I are a team. And as in any sport, someone has to lose, but as everyone knows, it's how you play the game that counts. When you look at yourself in the mirror and know that you've done your best, you will truly be at peace.

Notes

Foreword

1. American Lung Association. Lung Cancer Fact Sheet. Available at: http://www.lung.org/lung-health-and-diseases/lung-disease-lookup/lung-cancer/learn-about-lung-cancer/lung-cancer-fact-sheet.html

Chapter 1

1. Rochester DF. The diaphragm: contractile properties and fatigue. *Journal of Clinical Investigation*. 1985;75(5):1397–1402.

2. Tour the respiratory system. Verywell.com. http://copd.about.com/od/copd/ig/Respiratory-System.–RW/Diaphragm.htm

3. Hanson R. Relaxed and contented: activating the parasympathetic wing of your nervous system. http://www.wisebrain.org/ParasympatheticNS.pdf

4. Joy O. The science behind positive thinking your way to success. CNN.com. http://www.cnn.com/2013/10/11/business/the-science-behind-positive-thinking

5. Zmijewski C. Activate the parasympathetic nervous system to improve recovery. PTontheNet.com. http://www.ptonthenet.com/articles/activate-the-parasympathetic-nervous-system-to-improve-recovery-3910

6. Pal GK, Agarwal A, Karthik S, Pal P, Nanda N. Slow yogic breathing through right and left nostril influences sympathovagal balance, heart rate variability, and cardiovascular risks in young adults. *North American Journal of Medical Sciences*. 2014;6(3):145–151. doi:10.4103/1947-2714.128477

7. Weil A. The art and science of breathing. http://www.drweil.com/drw/u/ART02039/the-art-and-science-of-breathing.html

8. Kramer H, Groen HJM. Current Concepts in the Mediastinal Lymph Node Staging of Nonsmall Cell Lung Cancer. *Annals of Surgery.* 2003;238(2):180–188. doi:10.1097/01.SLA.0000081086.37779.1a

9. American Physiological Society. Lungs Try to Repair Damaged Elastic Fibers. *Science Daily.* Available at: www.sciencedaily.com/releases/2006 /11/061103083537.htm

10. Paxton J. *An Introduction to the Study of Human Anatomy*, Volume 2. Boston: William D. Ticknor, 1837; p. 39.

Chapter 2

1. Berger, NA, Savvides P, Koroukian SM, et al. Cancer in the Elderly. *Transactions of the American Clinical and Climatological Association.* 2006;117:147–156.

2. National Cancer Institute. Cancer types. http://www.cancer.gov/types

3. American Cancer Society. Cancer facts and figures 2015. http://www .cancer.org/acs/groups/content/@editorial/documents/document/acspc-04 4552.pdf

4. Chilkov N. What causes cancer? Genetics & environment: the perfect storm. The Huffington Post. http://www.huffingtonpost.com/nalini-chilkov /environments-cancer_b_901210.html

5. American Cancer Society. Genetics and cancer. http://www.cancer.org /cancer/cancercauses/geneticsandcancer/genetictesting/genetic-testing-intro

6. Sharma S, Kelly TK, Jones PA. Epigenetics in cancer. *Carcinogenesis.* 2010;31(1):27–36. doi:10.1093/carcin/bgp220

7. Larsen JE, Minna JD. Molecular biology of lung cancer: clinical implications. *Clinics in Chest Medicine.* 2011;32(4):703–740. doi:10.1016/j. ccm.2011.08.003.

8. Luo SY, Lam DCL. Oncogenic driver mutations in lung cancer. *Translational Respiratory Medicine* 2013;1:6. doi:10.1186/2213-0802-1-6

9. Zhao J, Xiong J. Advances on driver oncogenes of non-small cell lung cancer. 2015;18(1):42–47. doi: 10.3779/j.issn.1009-3419.2015.01.07

10. American Cancer Society. Genes and cancer. http://www.cancer.org /acs/groups/cid/documents/webcontent/002550-pdf.pdf.

11. Pfeifer GP, Denissenko MF, Olivier M, et al. Tobacco smoke carcinogens, DNA damage and p53 mutations in smoking-associated cancers. *Oncogene.* 2002;21:7435–7451. doi:10.1038/sj.onc.1205803

12. Zhu Z, Aref AR, Cohoon TJ, et al. Inhibition of *KRAS*-driven tumorigenicity by interruption of an autocrine cytokine circuit. *Cancer Discovery.* http://cancerdiscovery.aacrjournals.org/content/4/4/452.abstract #cited-by

13. National Cancer Institute. Tumor grade. http://www.cancer.gov /about-cancer/diagnosis-staging/prognosis/tumor-grade-fact-sheet

14. Hanahan D, Weinberg RA. The hallmarks of cancer. *Cell.* 2000;100(1):57–70. PMID: 10647931

Chapter 3

1. Centers for Disease Control and Prevention. National Center for Health Statistics. CDC WONDER On-line Database, compiled from Compressed Mortality File 1999–2012 Series 20 No. 2R, 2014.

2. World Cancer Report 2014. http://www.who.int/mediacentre/fact sheets/fs297/en

3. Smith EA, Malone RE. "Everywhere the soldier will be": wartime tobacco promotion in the US Military. *American Journal of Public Health.* 2009;99(9):1595–1602. doi:10.2105/AJPH.2008.152983

4. Furrukh M. Tobacco smoking and lung cancer: perception-changing facts. *Sultan Qaboos University Medical Journal.* 2013;13(3):345–358.

5. U.S. Department of Health, Education, and Welfare, Public Health Service. *Smoking and Health: Report of the Advisory Committee to the Surgeon General of the Public Health Service.* https://profiles.nlm.nih.gov/ps/access/NNBBMQ.pdf

6. Office on Smoking and Health. Patterns of tobacco use among women and girls. In *Women and Smoking: A Report of the Surgeon General.* Atlanta, GA: Centers for Disease Control and Prevention; 2001: chapter 2. Available at: http://www.ncbi.nlm.nih.gov/books/NBK44311

7. International Agency for Research on Cancer. GLOBOCAN 2012: Estimated cancer incidence, mortality and prevalence worldwide in 2012. http://globocan.iarc.fr/Default.aspx

8. Clague J, Reynolds P, Henderson KD, et al. Menopause hormone therapy and lung cancer-specific mortality following diagnosis. The California Teaches Study. *PLoS One.* July 31, 2014. http://journals.plos.org/plosone/article?id=10.1371%2Fjournal.pone.0103735

9. Berger AH, Pandolfi PP. Cancer Susceptibility Syndromes. In: DeVita VT, Lawrence TS, Rosenberg SA, eds. *DeVita, Hellman, and Rosenberg's Cancer: Principles and Practice of Oncology.* 8th ed. Philadelphia: Lippincott Williams & Wilkins; 2011:161–172. http://www.cancer.org/cancer/cancer causes/genetics andcancer/heredity-and-cancer

10. Hoang T, Dahlberg SE, Sandler AB, et al. Prognostic models to predict survival in non-small cell lung cancer patients treated with first-line paclitaxel and carboplatin with or without bevacizumab. *Journal of Thoracic Oncology.* 2012;7(9):1361–1368. doi:10.1097/JTO.0b013e318260e106

11. American Cancer Society. Lung cancer (non–small cell). http://www.cancer.org/acs/groups/cid/documents/webcontent/003115-pdf.pdf

12. Former smokers and cancer risk. OncoLink. http://www.oncolink.org/risk/article.cfm?id=22

13. Cancer Research UK. Smoking facts and evidence. http://www.cancerresearchuk.org/about-cancer/causes-of-cancer/smoking-and-cancer/smoking-facts-and-evidence

14. Stead LF, Perera R, Bullen C, et al. Nicotine replacement therapy for smoking cessation. *Cochrane Database Systematic Reviews.* 2012;11: CD000146. doi: 10.1002/14651858.CD000146.pub4

15. National Cancer Institute. Secondhand smoke and cancer. http://www.cancer.gov/about-cancer/causes-prevention/risk/tobacco/second-hand-smoke-fact-sheet

16. National Cancer Institute. Radon and cancer. http://www.cancer.gov/about-cancer/causes-prevention/risk/substances/radon/radon-fact-sheet

17. Martinez VD, Vucic EA, Becker-Santso DD, et al. Arsenic exposure and the induction of human cancers. *Journal of Toxicology.* 2011;(2011): Article ID 431287 (http://dx.doi.org/10.1155/2011/431287)

18. Halasova E, Matakova T, Kavcova E, Singliar A. Human lung cancer and hexavalent chromium exposure. *Neuroendocrinology Letters.* 2009;30 (suppl 1):182–185.

19. Grimsrud TK, Berge SR, Haldorsen T, Andersen A. Exposure to different forms of nickel and risk of lung cancer. *American Journal of Epidemiolgoy.* 2002;156(12):1123–1132 doi:10.1093/aje/kwf165.

20. Miller BG, Doust E, Cherrie JW, Hurley JF. Lung cancer mortality and exposure to polycyclic aromatic hydrocarbons in British coke oven workers. *BMC Public Health* 2013, 13:962 doi:10.1186/1471-2458-13-962

21. Shen H, Tao S, Liu J, et al. Global lung cancer risk from PAH exposure highly depends on emission sources and individual susceptibility. *Scientific Reports.* 2014;4: article 6561. http://www.nature.com/articles/srep06561

22. Cell division and cancer. Scitable by Nature Education. http://www.nature.com/scitable/topicpage/cell-division-and-cancer-14046590

23. Stratton MR, Campbell PJ, Futreal PA. The cancer genome. *Nature.* 2009;458(7239):719–724. doi:10.1038/nature07943

24. Cancer Treatment and Survivorship Facts and Figures. 2014–2015. http://www.cancer.org/acs/groups/content/@research/documents/document/acspc-042801.pdf

25. Ershler WB, Longo DL. Aging and cancer: issues of basic and clinical science. *Journal of the National Cancer Institute.* 1997:89(20):1489–1497. doi: 10.1093/jnci/89.20.1489; http://jnci.oxfordjournals.org/content/89/20/1489.full

26. New study looks at growth rates of lung cancers found by ct screening. *Radiological Society of North America*, March 27, 2012. https://www2.rsna.org/timssnet/media/pressreleases/pr_target.cfm?ID=598.

27. K Pantel. Detection and clinical importance of micrometastatic disease. *Journal of the National Cancer Institute.* 1999;91(13):1113–1124. doi: 10.1093/jnci/91.13.1113; http://jnci.oxfordjournals.org/content/91/13/1113.full

28. Rehktman N, Ang DC, Sima CS, et al. Immunohistochemical algorithm for differentiation of lung adenocarcinoma and squamous cell carcinoma based on large series of whole-tissue sections with validation in small specimens. *Modern Pathology.* 2011;24(10):1348–1359. doi: 10.1038/modpathol.2011.92

29. Tan WT, Huq Syed. Non–small cell lung cancer. http://emedicine .medscape.com/article/279960-overview

30. Lewis DR, Check DP, Caporaso NE, et al. US lung cancer trends by histologic type. *Cancer.* 2014;120(18):2883–2892. doi: 10.1002/cncr.28749

31. Tan WW. Non–small cell lung cancer. http://emedicine.medscape .com/article/279960-overview

32. Ibid.

33. Travis WD, Brambilla E, Müller-Hermelink HK, Harris CC. Tumors of the lungs. From *Pathology & Genetics: Tumours of the Lungs, Thymus, Pleura and Heart.* http://www.iarc.fr/en/publications/pdfs-online/pat-gen /bb10/bb10-chap1.pdf

34. Takei H, Asamura H, Maeshima A, et al. Large cell neuroendocrine carcinoma of the lung: a clinicopathologic study of eighty-seven cases. *Journal of Thoracic and Cardiovascular Surgery.* 2002;124(2):285–292.

35. Parsons A, Daley A, Begh R, Aveyard P. Influence of smoking cessation after diagnosis of early stage lung cancer on prognosis: systematic review of observational studies with meta-analysis. *BMJ.* 2010;340:b556.

36. Janne PA, Freidlin B, Saxman S, et al. Twenty-five years of clinical research for patients with limited-stage small cell lung carcinoma in North America. *Cancer.* 2002;95(7):1528–1538.

37. American Cancer Society. Malignant mesothelioma. http://www.caring forcarcinoid.org/neuroendocrine-cancer/carcinoid-cancer-1

38. Porpodis K, Zarogoulidis P, Boutsikou E, et al. Malignant pleural mesothelioma: current and future perspectives. *Journal of Thoracic Disease.* 2013;5(suppl 4): S397–S406.

Chapter 4

1. National Lung Screening Trial Research Team. Reduced lung-cancer mortality with low-dose computed tomographic screening. *New England Journal of Medicine.* 2011;365(5):395–409. doi: 10.1056/NEJMoa1102873

2. Mckee A, Salner A. A cancer battle we can win. *New York Times,* September 21, 2014.

3. Providing Guidance on Lung Cancer Screening to Patients and Physicians: An Update from the American Lung Association Lung Cancer Screening Committee. April 15, 2013. http://www.lung.org/assets/documents /lung-cancer/lung-cancer-screening-report.pdf

4. American College of Radiology. Study confirms CT lung cancer screening is cost effective: full Medicare coverage should follow. ScienceDaily. http://www.sciencedaily.com/releases/2014/09/140902144049.htm

5. Pyenson BS, Sander MS, Jiang Y, et al. An actuarial analysis shows that offering lung cancer screening as an insurance benefit would save lives at relatively low cost. *Health Affairs.* 2012;31(4):770–779. doi: 10.1377/ hlthaff.2011.0814

6. Mitchell ED, Pickwell-Smith B, Macleod U. Risk factors for emergency presentation with lung and colorectal cancers: a systematic review. *BMJ Open* 2015;5:e006965 doi:10.1136/bmjopen-2014-006965

7. Ferrell B, Koczywas M, Grannis F, Harrington A. Palliative care in lung cancer. *Surgical Clinics of North America.* 2011;91(2):403–417. doi:10.1016/j.suc.2010.12.003

8. Tan WW. Non–small cell lung cancer clinical presentation. http://emedicine.medscape.com/article/279960-clinical

9. Ammanagi AS, Dombale VD, Miskin AT, et al. Sputum cytology in suspected cases of carcinoma of lung (sputum cytology a poor man's bronchoscopy!). *Lung India.* 2012;29(1):19–23.

10. Grunnet M, Sorensen JB. Carcinoembryonic antigen (CEA) as a tumor marker in lung cancer. *Lung Cancer.* 2012 May;76(2):138–143. doi: 10.1016/j.lungcan.2011.11.012

11. The National Lung Screening Trial Research Team. Reduced lung-cancer mortality with low-dose computed tomographic screening. *New England Journal of Medicine.* 2011;365:395–409 doi: 10.1056/NEJMoa 1102873

12. National Heart, Lung, and Blood Institute. What is bronchoscopy? http://www.nhlbi.nih.gov/health/health-topics/topics/bron

13. National Comprehensive Cancer Network. Cancer staging guide. http://www.nccn.org/patients/resources/diagnosis/staging.aspx

14. Ibid.

15. Ibid.

16. Detterbeck FC, Boffa DJ, Tanoue LT. The new lung cancer staging system. *Chest.* 2009;136(1):260–271.

17. Mirsadraee S, Oswal D, Alizadeh Y, et al. The 7th lung cancer TNM classification and staging system: review of the changes and implications. *World Journal of Radiology.* 2012;4(4):128–134. doi:10.4329/wjr.v4.i4.128

18. Ready NE, Pang HH, Gu L, et al. Chemotherapy with or without maintenance sunitinib for untreated extensive-stage small-cell lung cancer: a randomized, double-blind, placebo-controlled Phase II study-CALGB 30504 (Alliance). *J Clin Oncol.* 2015;33(15):166.

Chapter 5

1. National Collaborating Centre for Cancer. Treatment with curative intent for NSCLC. In *The Diagnosis and Treatment of Lung Cancer* (Update) (NICE Clinical Guidelines No. 121.) Cardiff, United Kingdom: National Collaborating Centre for Cancer; 2011. http://www.ncbi.nlm.nih.gov/books /NBK99025

2. Sarcoma, soft tissue: treatment options. Cancer.Net. http://www .cancer.net/cancer-types/sarcoma-soft-tissue/treatment-options

3. National Cancer Institute. NCI Dictionary of Cancer Terms. http:// www.cancer.gov/publications/dictionaries/cancer-terms?cdrid=346513

4. Jessy T. Immunity over inability: the spontaneous regression of cancer. *Journal of Natural Science, Biology, and Medicine.* 2011;2(1):43–49. doi:10.4103/0976-9668.82318

5. O'Regan B, Hirschberg C. *Spontaneous Remission: An Annotated Bibliography.* Petaluma, CA: Institute of Noetic Sciences; 1993.

6. Lenzer J. The body can stave off terminal cancer—sometimes. *Discover,* September 2007. http://discovermagazine.com/2007/sep/the-body-can-stave -off-terminal-cancer-sometimes

7. Turner KA. *Radical Remissions: Surviving Cancer Against All Odds.* New York: HarperOne; 2014.

8. Nelson R. Radical remissions: cancer patients who defy the odds. July 8, 2014. http://www.medscape.com/viewarticle/827945

9. Burmeis BH, Henderson MA, Ainslie J, et al. Adjuvant radiotherapy versus observation alone for patients at risk of lymph-node field relapse after therapeutic lymphadenectomy for melanoma: a randomised trial. *Lancet Oncology.* 2012;13(6):589–597. doi: 10.1016/S1470-2045(12) 70138-9

10. R. Thomas, James N, Guerrero D, et al. Hypofractionated radiotherapy as palliative treatment in poor prognosis patients with high grade glioma. *Radiotherapy and Oncology.* 1994;33(2):113–116. doi:10.1016/ 0167-8140(94)90064-7.

11. Zelefsky MJ, Fuks Z, Happersett L, et al. Clinical experience with intensity modulated radiation therapy (IMRT) in prostate cancer. *Radiotherapy and Oncology.* 2000;55(3):241–249.

12. Intensity-Modulated Radiation Therapy (IMRT). RadiologyInfo.org. June 15, 2015. http://www.radiologyinfo.org/en/info.cfm?pg=imrt

13. Kim DW, Chung K, Chung WK, et al. Risk of secondary cancers from scattered radiation during intensity-modulated radiotherapies for hepatocellular carcinoma. *Radiation Oncology (London, England).* 2014;9:109. doi:10.1186/1748-717X-9-109

14. Cossman PH. Advances in image-guided radiotherapy—the future is in motion. *US Oncology Review.* 2005;1(1):36–40.

15. Chang, Li-Fen L. et al. High dose rate afterloading intraluminal brachytherapy in malignant airway obstruction of lung cancer. *International Journal of Radiation, Oncology, Biology and Physics.* 1994;28(3):589–596. http://dx.doi.org/10.1016/0360-3016(94)90183-X

16. American Cancer Society. External radiation. In *A Guide to Radiation Therapy.* Updated 6/30/2015. http://www.cancer.org/treatment/treatment sandsideeffects/treatmenttypes/radiation/understandingradiationtherapy aguideforpatientsandfamilies/understanding-radiation-therapy-external -radiation-therapy

17. Zhao Y, Qi G, Yin G. A clinical study of lung cancer dose calculation accuracy with Monte Carlo simulation. *Radiation Oncology.* 2014;9:287. doi: 10.1186/s13014-014-0287-2. http://www.ncbi.nlm.nih.gov/pubmed /25511623

18. Salvo N, Barnes E, van Draanen J, et al. Prophylaxis and management of acute radiation-induced skin reactions: a systematic review of the literature. *Current Oncology.* 2010;17(4):94–112.

19. Sandy B. Esophagitis during lung cancer treatment. *Oncolink.* http://www.oncolink.org/experts/article.cfm?id=2546

20. Mehta V. Radiation pneumonitis and pulmonary fibrosis in non-small-cell lung cancer: pulmonary function, prediction, and prevention. *International Journal of Radiation, Oncology, Biology and Physics.* 2005;63(1):5–24. http://www.ncbi.nlm.nih.gov/pubmed/15963660

21. Agrawal S. Clinical relevance of radiation pneumonitis in breast cancers. *South Asian Journal of Cancer.* 2013;2(1):19–20. doi:10.4103/2278 330X.105885

22. Bello S, Menéndez R, Torres A, et al. Tobacco smoking increases the risk for death from pneumococcal pneumonia. *Chest.* 2014;146(4):1029–1037. doi:10.1378/chest.13-2853

23. Wallace WA, Fitch PM, Simpson AJ, Howie SE. Inflammation-associated remodelling and fibrosis in the lung—a process and an end point. *International Journal of Experimental Pathology.* 2007;88(2):103–110. doi:10.1111/j.1365-2613.2006.00515.x

24. University of Texas M. D. Anderson Cancer Center. Pioneers in the fight against "The Big One": Proton therapy for lung cancer. *ScienceDaily.* http://www.sciencedaily.com/releases/2013/11/131112141241.htm

25. Chang JY, et al. Significant reduction of normal tissue dose by proton radiotherapy compared with three-dimensional conformal or intensity-modulated radiation therapy in Stage I or Stage III non–small-cell lung cancer. *International Journal of Radiation, Oncology, Biology and Physics.* 2006;65(4):1087–1096.

26. Press Release: Proton therapy's fight against lung cancer: M.D. Anderson physicians pioneer the fight led by Dr. James Cox, Keynote Speaker at NPC2014 in Washington D.C. Released: 11/12/2013. The National Association for Proton Therapy. http://www.proton-therapy.org/fight_against_lung_cancer.html

27. Karakayali FY. Surgical and interventional management of complications caused by acute pancreatitis. *World Journal of Gastroenterology* 2014;20(37):13412–13423. doi:10.3748/wjg.v20.i37.13412

28. Ibrahim AM, Hughes TG, Thumma JR, Dimick JB. Association of hospital critical access status with surgical outcomes among medicare beneficiaries. *JAMA.* 2016;315(19)2095.

29. Cooper MA, Hutfless S, Segeve DL, et al. Hospital level under-utilization of minimally invasive surgery in the United States: retrospective review. *BMJ* 2014;349:g4198. doi: http://dx.doi.org/10.1136/bmj.g4198

30. Narsule CK, Ebright MI, Fernando HC. Sublobar versus lobar resection: current status. *Cancer Journal.* 2011;17(1):23–27.

31. Travis W, Brambilla E, Noguchi M, et al. International Association for the Study of Lung Cancer/American Thoracic Society/European

Respiratory Society International Multidisciplinary Classification of Lung Adenocarcinoma. *Journal of Thoracic Oncology.* 2011;6(2):244–285.

32. Ruckdeschel JC, Greene J, Sommers KE, et al. Surgical complications causing dyspnea in cancer patients. In Kufe DW, Pollock RE, Weichselbaum RR, et al., eds. *Holland-Frei Cancer Medicine.* 6th ed. Hamilton, Canada: BC Decker; 2003. Available from: http://www.ncbi.nlm.nih.gov/books/NBK12774

33. Holgersson G, Bergström S, Ekman S. Radiosensitizing biological modifiers enhancing efficacy in non-small-cell lung cancer treated with radiotherapy. *Lung Cancer Management.* 2(4):251–255. http://www.future medicine.com/doi/abs/10.2217/lmt.13.25?journalCode=lmt

34. Koukourakis MI. Radiation damage and radioprotectants: new concepts in the era of molecular medicine. *British Journal of Radiology.* 2012;85(1012):313–330. doi:10.1259/bjr/16386034

35. National Cancer Institute. General Information About Small Cell Lung Cancer (SCLC). http://www.cancer.gov/types/lung/hp/small-cell-lung -treatment-pdq

36. JJ Mazeron, Scalliet P, Van Limbergen E, Lartigau E. Radiobiology of brachytherapy and the dose-rate effect. http://www.estro.org/binaries /content/assets/estro/about/gec-estro/handbook-of-brachytherapy/e -4-23072002-radiobiology-print_proc.pdf

37. Haslett K, Pöttgen C, Stuschke M, Faivre-Finn C. Hyperfractionated and accelerated radiotherapy in non-small cell lung cancer. *Journal of Thoracic Disease.* 2014;6(4):328–335. doi:10.3978/j.issn.2072-1439.2013. 11.06

38. Rosell R. Predicting response to chemotherapy with early-stage lung cancer. *Cancer Journal.* 2011;17:49–56. doi: 10.1097/PPO.0b013e31820 91fa3

39. Inhaled chemotherapy is most effective in lung cancer. *BioSpectrum: The Business of Bioscience.* June 13, 2013. http://www.biospectrumasia. com/biospectrum/news/190001/inhaled-chemotherapy-effective-lung -cancer.

40. Zarogoulidis P, Chatzaki E, Porpodis K, et al. Inhaled chemotherapy in lung cancer: future concept of nanomedicine. *International Journal of Nanomedicine.* 2012;7:1551–1572. doi:10.2147/IJN.S29997

41. Patient information: Non-small cell lung cancer treatment; stage IV cancer (Beyond the Basics). *Up-to-Date.* http://www.uptodate.com/contents /non-small-cell-lung-cancer-treatment-stage-iv-cancer-beyond-the-basics

42. Solomon BJ, Mok T, Dong-Wan K, et al. First-line crizotinib versus chemotherapy in *ALK*-positive lung cancer. *New England Journal of Medicine.* 2014;371:2167–2177. doi: 10.1056/NEJMoa1408440

43. Bisht M, Dhasmana DC, Bist SS. Angiogenesis: future of pharmaco-logical modulation. *Indian Journal of Pharmacology.* 2010;42(1):2–8. doi:10.4103/0253-7613.62395

44. Yoo SY, Kwon SM. Angiogenesis and its therapeutic opportunities. *Mediators of Inflammation,* 2013; article ID 127170. doi:10.1155/2013/127170

45. Thalidomide in small cell lung cancer: wrong drug or wrong disease? *Journal of the National Cancer Institute.* 2009;101(15):1034–1035. doi: 10.1093/jnci/djp208. http://jnci.oxfordjournals.org/content/101/15 /1034.full

46. Cohen MH, Gootenberg J, Keegan P, Pazdur R. FDA drug approval summary: bevacizumab (Avastin) plus carboplatin and paclitaxel as first-line treatment of advanced/metastatic recurrent nonsquamous non-small cell lung cancer. *Oncologist.* 2007;12(6):713–718. http://www.ncbi.nlm .nih.gov/pubmed/17602060

47. Marr AS, Ganti AK. Advanced lung cancer in the older patient: is there a role for bevacizumab? *Journal of Thoracic Disease.* 2012;4(6):629–630. doi: 10.3978/j.issn.2072-1439.2012.09.07

48. Mantanić D, Beg-Zec Z, Stojanović D, et al. Cytokines in patients with lung cancer. *Scandinavian Journal of Immunology.* 2003;57(2):173–178.

49. Wang Y. Monoclonal antibodies in lung cancer. *Expert Opinion on Biological Therapy.* 2013;13(2):209–226. doi: 10.1517/14712598.2012. 748742

50. Pastan I, Hassan R, FitzGerald DJ, Kreitman RJ. Immunotoxin treatment of cancer. *Annual Review of Medicine.* 2007;58:221–237.

51. Ehrlich D, Wang B, Lu W, et al. Intratumoral anti-HuD immunotoxin therapy for small cell lung cancer and neuroblastoma. *Journal of Hematology & Oncology.* 2014;7:91. doi:10.1186/s13045-014-0091-3

52. Ross H, Hart L, Swanson P, et al. A randomized, multicenter study to determine the safety and efficacy of the immunoconjugate SGN-15 plus docetaxel for the treatment of non-small cell lung carcinoma. *Lung Cancer.* 2006;54;69–77.

53. http://www.ascopost.com/issues/september-10,-2015/roswell-park -cancer-institute-partners-with-cuban-scientists-to-develop-lung-cancer -vaccine.

54. Neninger VE, de la Torre A, Osorio Rodriguez M, et al. Phase II randomized controlled trial of an epidermal growth factor vaccine in advanced non-small-cell lung cancer. *Journal of Clinical Oncology.* 2008;26(9):1452–1458. doi: 10.1200/JCO.2007.11.5980

55. Gomez A, Szabo L. "Cuban cancer vaccine3 to be tested in U.S. sparks a new scientific bond. *USA Today.* May 13, 2015. http://www.usatoday.com /story/news/2015/05/13/cuba-lung-cancer-vaccine-scientific-collabo ration/27241137

56. Theisen C. Chemoprevention: What's in a name? *Journal of the National Cancer Institute.* 2001;93:743.

57. Steward WP, Brown K. Cancer chemoprevention: a rapidly evolving field. *British Journal of Cancer.* 2013;109:1–7. doi:10.1038/bjc.2013.280

58. Fernando HC, De Hoyos A, Landreneau RJ, et al. Radiofrequency ablation for the treatment of non-small cell lung cancer in marginal surgical candidates. *Journal of Thoracic Cardiovascular Surgery.* 2005;129(3):639–644.

59. Inoue M, Nakatsuka S, Jinzaki M. Cryoablation of early-stage primary lung cancer. *BioMed Research International*. 2014; article ID 521691. doi:10.1155/2014/521691

60. Vogl TJ, Shafinaderi M, Zangos S, et al. Regional chemotherapy of the lung: transpulmonary chemoembolization in malignant lung tumors. *Seminars in Interventional Radiology*. 2013;30(2):176–184. doi:10.1055/s -0033-1342959

61. Giovannetti E, Toffarlorio F, De Pas T, Peters GJ. Pharmacogenetics of conventional chemotherapy in non-small-cell lung cancer: a changing landscape? *Pharmacogenomics*. 2012;13(9):1073–1086. doi: 10.2217/pgs.12.91

62. Creelan BC. Update on immune checkpoint inhibitors in lung cancer. *Cancer Control: Journal of the Moffitt Cancer Center*. 2014. https://moffitt .org/File%20Library/Main%20Nav/Research%20and%20Clinical%20 Trials/Cancer%20Control%20Journal/v21n1/80.pdf

63. Cris MG. Two decades of lung cancer advances. Medscape Oncology. http://www.medscape.com/viewarticle/844652

Chapter 6

1. Ratson G. *The Meaning of Health: The Experience of a Lifetime*. Victoria, Canada: Trafford; 2006.

2. Hudson RP. *Disease and Its Control*. Westport, CT: Praeger; 1983:78.

3. Complementary and alternative medicine. MedicineNet. http://www .medicinenet.com/alternative_medicine/page2.htm

4. Complementary and Alternative Medicine (CAM). Medicine.net. http://www.medicinenet.com/alternative_medicine/page2.htm

5. Services, 2016.

6. https://www.acatoday.org/level2_css.cfm?T1ID=13&T2ID=61

7. Vickers AJ. Independent replication of pre-clinical research in homeopathy: a systematic review. *Forschende Komplementarmedezin*. 1999;6: 311–320.

8. Brien S, Prescott P, Owen D, Lewith G. How do homeopaths make decisions? An exploratory study of inter-rater reliability and intuition in the decision making process. *Homeopathy*. 2004;93(3):125–131.

9. Clark IA. The advent of the cytokine storm. *Immunology and Cell Biology*. 2007;85:271–273; doi:10.1038/sj.icb.7100062

10. Stuckey HL, Nobel J. The connection between art, healing, and public health: a review of current literature. *American Journal of Public Health*. 2010;100(2):254–263.

11. Welling A. What is dance/movement therapy? American Dance Therapy Association. http://www.adta.org

12. Shabanloei R. Effects of music therapy on pain and anxiety in patients undergoing bone marrow biopsy and aspiration. *AORN Journal*. 2010;91(6):746–751. doi: 10.1016/j.aorn.2010.04.001

13. Macmillan Cancer Support. Dramatherapy—a psychological therapy. Winter 2012. http://www.macmillan.org.uk/Aboutus/Healthandsocial careprofessionals/Newsandupdates/MacVoice/MacVoiceWinter2012 /Dramatherapy–apsychologicaltherapy.aspx

14. Puetz TW, Morley CA, Herring MP. Effects of creative arts therapies on psychological symptoms and quality of life in patients with cancer. *JAMA Internal Medicine.* 2013;173(11):960–969. doi:10.1001/jamainternmed. 2013.836

15. Kerson C. A proposed multisite double-blind randomized clinical trial of neurofeedback for ADHD: need, rationale, and strategy. *Journal of Attention Disorders.* 2013;17:420–436.

16. Sonuga-Barke EJS, et al., Nonpharmacological interventions for ADHD: systematic review and meta-analyses of randomized controlled trials of dietary and psychological treatments. *American Journal of Psychiatry.* 2013;170:275–289. http://dx.doi.org/10.1176/appi.ajp.2012.12070991

17. Montgomery GH, et al. Hypnosis for cancer care: over 200 years young. *CA: A Cancer Journal for Clinicians.* 2013;63(1):31–34. doi: 10.3322/caac.21165

18. Ernst E. Massage therapy for cancer palliation and supportive care: a systematic review of randomised clinical trials. *Support Care Cancer.* 2009;17(4):333–337.

19. Cancer Research UK. Massage (manual lymphatic drainage) treatment for lymphoedema. http://www.cancerresearchuk.org/about-cancer /coping-with-cancer/coping-physically/lymphoedema/treating-lymphoe dema/massage-mldfor-lymphoedema

20. Neuromuscular massage therapy. Spine-health. http://www .spine-health.com/wellness/massage-therapy/neuromuscular-massage -therapy

21. Long AF. The effectiveness of shiatsu: findings from a cross-European, prospective observational study. *Journal of Alternative and Complementary Medicine.* 2008;14(8):921–930. doi: 10.1089/acm.2008.0085

22. Robinson N, Lorenc A, Liao X. The evidence for shiatsu: a systematic review of shiatsu and acupressure. *BMC Complementary and Alternative Medicine.* 2011;11:88. doi: 10.1186/1472-6882-11-88

23. Larkey LK, Roe DJ, Weihs KL, et al. Randomized controlled trial of Qigong/Tai Chi Easy on cancer-related fatigue in breast cancer survivors. *Annals of Behavior Medicine* 2015;49(2):165–176. doi: 10.1007/s12160 -014-9645-4

24. Levine ME, Suarez JA, Bradhorst S, et al. Low protein intake is associated with a major reduction in IGF-1, cancer, and overall mortality in the 65 and younger but not older population. *Cell Metabolism.* 2014;19(3):407–417.

25. What are the best vitamins for cancer patients? Dana-Farber Cancer Institute. December 14, 2011. http://blog.dana-farber.org/insight/2011/12 /what-are-the-best-vitamins-for-cancer-patients

26. Martinez ME, et al. Dietary supplements and cancer prevention: balancing potential benefits against proven harms. *Journal of the National Cancer Institute.* 2012;104(10):732–739. doi: 10.1093/jnci/djs195

27. Parker-Pop T. Despite risks, vitamins popular with cancer patients. *New York Times.* February 6, 2008. http://well.blogs.nytimes.com/2008 /02/06/despite-risks-vitamins-popular-with-cancer-patients/?_r=0

28. Velicer CM, Ulrich CM. Vitamin and mineral supplement use among US adults after cancer diagnosis: a systematic review. *Journal of Clinical Oncology.* 2008;26(4):665–673. doi: 10.1200/JCO.2007.13.5905

29. Goralczyk R. Beta-carotene and lung cancer in smokers: review of hypotheses and status of research. *Nutrition and Cancer.* 2009;61(6):767–774. doi: 10.1080/01635580903285155

30. Wright ME, Groshong SD, Husgafvel-Pursiainen K, et al. Effects of β-carotene supplementation on molecular markers of lung carcinogenesis in male smokers. *Cancer Prevention Research.* 2010;3(6):745–752. doi:10.1158/ 1940-6207.CAPR-09-0107

31. Sayin VI, Ibrahim MX, Larsson E, et al. Antioxidants accelerate lung cancer progression in mice. *Science Translational Medicine.* 2014;29;6(221): 221ra15. doi: 10.1126/scitranslmed.3007653

32. National Cancer Institute. Lung cancer prevention. http://www .cancer.gov/types/lung/hp/lung-prevention-pdq

33. Luo J, Shen L, Zheng D. Association between vitamin C intake and lung cancer: a dose-response meta-analysis. *Scientific Reports.* 2014;4: article 6161. doi:10.1038/srep06161

34. Fritz H, Kennedy D, Fergusson D, et al. Selenium and lung cancer: a systematic review and meta analysis. *PLoS ONE.* 2011;6(11):e26259. doi:10.1371/journal.pone.0026259.

35. Prasad AS. Zinc in human health: effect of zinc on immune cells. *Molecular Medicine.* 2008;14(5-6):353–357. doi:10.2119/2008-00033. Prasad

36. Lockwood K, Moesgaard S, Folkers. Partial and complete regression of breast cancer in patients in relation to dosage of coenzyme Q10. *Biochemistry and Biophysics Research Communications.* 1994;199(3):1504 –1508.

37. Glinsky VV, Raz A. Modified citrus pectin anti-metastatic properties: one bullet, multiple targets. *Carbohydrate Research.* 2009;344(14):1788–1791. doi:10.1016/j.carres.2008.08.038

38. Hensley CT, Wasti AT, DeBerardinis RJ. Glutamine and cancer: cell biology, physiology, and clinical opportunities. *The Journal of Clinical Investigation.* 2013;123(9):3678–3684. doi:10.1172/JCI69600.

39. Jin Z-Y, Wu M, Han R-Q, et al. Raw garlic consumption as a protective factor for lung cancer, a population-based case-control study in a Chinese population. *Cancer Prevention Research.* 2013;6(7):711–718. doi:10.1158/1940-6207.CAPR-13-0015

40. Blask DE, Sauer LA, Dauchy RT. Melatonin as a chronobiotic/anticancer agent: Cellular, biochemical, and molecular mechanisms of action and their implications for circadian-based cancer therapy. *Current Topics in Medicinal Chemistry.* 2002;2:113–132.

41. Blask DE, Dauchy RT, Brainard GC, Hanifin JP. Circadian stage-dependent inhibition of human breast cancer metabolism and growth by the nocturnal melatonin signal: consequences of its disruption by light at night in rats and women. *Integrative Cancer Therapy.* 2009;8(4):347–353. doi: 10.1177/1534735409352320

42. Brown AC. Anticancer activity of *Morinda citrifolia* (noni) fruit: a review. *Phytotherapy Research.* 2012;26(10):1427–1440. doi: 10.1002/ptr.4595

43. Trock BJ, Hilakivi-Clarke L, Clarke R. Meta-analysis of soy intake and breast cancer risk. *Journal of the National Cancer Institute.* 2006;98(7): 459–471. doi:10.1093/jnci/djj102

44. National Cancer Institute. Selected Vegetables/Sun's Soup. http://www.cancer.gov/about-cancer/treatment/cam/patient/suns-soup-pdq

45. Blaszyk A. Taking stock of bone broth: sorry, no cure-all here. http://www.npr.org/sections/thesalt/2015/02/10/384948585/taking-stock-of-bone-broth-sorry-no-cure-all-here

46. Rennard BO, Ertl RF, Gossman GL, et al. Chicken soup inhibits neutrophil chemotaxis in vitro. *Chest.* 2000;118(4):1150–1157.

47. Friedman LF. Here's why juicing is wasteful and unnecessary. *Business Insider.* June 20, 2016. http://www.businessinsider.com/juicing-and-juice-fasts-are-unnecessary-2016-6

48. Jia XH, Yin BH, Li JC. Effect of astragalus injection on U937 leukemia cells proliferation and apoptosis and relevant molecular mechanisms [in Chinese]. *Zhongguo Dang Dai Er Ke Za Zhi.* 2013;15(12):1128–1133

49. Guo L, Bai SP, Zhao L, Wang XH. Astragalus polysaccharide injection integrated with vinorelbine and cisplatin for patients with advanced non-small cell lung cancer: effects on quality of life and survival. *Medical Oncology.* 2012;29(3):1656–1662. doi: 10.1007/s12032-011-0068-9

50. Huang XY, Zhang SZ, Wang WX. Enhanced antitumor efficacy with combined administration of astragalus and pterostilbene for melanoma. *Asian Pacific Journal of Cancer Prevention.* 2014;15(3):1163–1169.

51. ConsumerLab. https://www.consumerlab.com

52. He H, Zhou X, Wang Q, Zhao Y. Does the course of astragalus-containing Chinese herbal prescriptions and radiotherapy benefit to non-small-cell lung cancer treatment: a meta-analysis of randomized trials. *Evidence-based Complementary and Alternative Medicine.* 2013;2013: 426207. doi:10.1155/2013/426207

53. Chan YS, Cheng LN, Wu JH, et al. A review of the pharmacological effects of *Arctium lappa* (burdock). *Inflammopharmacology.* 2011;19(5): 245–254.

54. Ferracane R, Graziani G, Gallo M, Fogliano V, Ritieni A. Metabolic profile of the bioactive compounds of burdock seeds, roots and leaves. *Journal of Pharmaceutical and Biomedical Analysis*. 2010;51(2):399–404.

55. Henning SM, Niu Y, Lee NH, et al. Bioavailability and antioxidant activity of tea flavonols after consumption of green tea, black tea, or a green tea extract supplement. *American Journal of Clinical Nutrition* 2004; 80(6):1558–1564.

56. Lambert JD, Yang CS. Mechanisms of cancer prevention by tea constituents. *Journal of Nutrition*. 2003;133(10):3262S–3267S.

57. Henning SM, Wang P, Heber D. Chemopreventive effects of tea in prostate cancer: green tea vs. black tea. *Molecular Nutrition & Food Research*. 2011;55(6):905–920. doi:10.1002/mnfr.201000648

58. Omar HR, Komarova I, El-Ghonemi M, et al. Licorice abuse: time to send a warning message. *Therapeutic Advances in Endocrinology and Metabolism*. 2012;3(4):125–138. doi: 10.1177/2042018812454322

59. Song NR, Lee E, Byun S, et al. Isoangustone A, a novel licorice compound, inhibits cell proliferation by targeting PI3K, MKK4, and MKK7 in human melanoma. *Cancer Prevention Research*. 2013;6(12):1293–1303. doi: 10.1158/1940-6207.CAPR-13-0134

60. Siegel AB, Stebbing J. Milk thistle: early seeds of potential. *The Lancet Oncology*. 2013;14(10):929–930. doi:10.1016/S1470-2045(13) 70414-5.

61. Shishodia S, Chaturvedi MM, Aggarwal BB. Role of curcumin in cancer therapy. *Current Problems in Cancer*. 2007;31(4):243–305.

62. Tumeric in Integrative Medicine. Source: Memorial Sloan Cancer Center. https://www.mskcc.org/cancer-care/integrative-medicine/herbs/tur meric. See also Moghaddam SJ, Barta P, Mirabolfathinejad SG, et al. Curcumin inhibits COPD-like airway inflammation and lung cancer progression in mice. *Carcinogenesis*. 2009;30(11):1949–1956. doi:10.1093/carcin/bgp229

63. Somasundaram S, Edmund NA, Moore DT, et al. Dietary curcumin inhibits chemotherapy-induced apoptosis in models of human breast cancer. *Cancer Research*. 2002;62:3868–3875.

64. Lv J, Qi L, Yu C, et al. Consumption of spicy foods and total and cause specific mortality: population based cohort study. *BMJ*. 2015;351:h3942.

65. Liao G-S, Apaya MK, Shyur L-F. Herbal medicine and acupuncture for breast cancer palliative care and adjuvant therapy. *Evidence-Based Complementary and Alternative Medicine*, 2013, Article ID 437948. doi:10.1155/2013/437948

Chapter 7

1. Institute of Medicine and National Academy of Engineering Roundtable on Value & Science-Driven Health Care. Healthcare System

Complexities, Impediments, and Failures. In *Engineering a Learning Healthcare System: A Look at the Future: Workshop Summary.* Washington, DC: National Academies Press; 2011: chap. 3. http://www.ncbi.nlm.nih.gov/books/NBK61963

2. Miller SA. Polls finds many confused about ObamaCare. *New York Post.* December 13, 2013. http://nypost.com/2013/12/13/poll-finds-many-confused-about-obamacare

3. Claxton G, Rae M, Panchal N, et al. Health benefits in 2015: stable trends in the employer market [published September 2015 online ahead of print]. *Health Affairs.* doi:10.1377/hlthaff.2015.0885

4. CancerCare. Your health care team: your doctor is only the beginning." CancerCare Fact Sheet. http://www.cancer.org/treatment/findingandpayingfortreatment/choosingyourtreatmentteam/health-professionals-associated-with-cancer-care See also: American Cancer Society. Health professionals associated with cancer care. In Choosing Your Cancer Care Team. http://www.cancer.org/treatment/findingandpayingfortreatment/choosingyourtreatmentteam/health-professionals-associated-with-cancer-care

5. Gaga, M, Powell, CA, Schraufnage, DE, et al. An official American Thoracic Society/European Respiratory Society Statement: The role of the pulmonologist in the diagnosis and management of lung cancer. http://www.cancer.org/treatment/findingandpayingfortreatment/choosingyourtreatmentteam/health-professionals-associated-with-cancer-care

6. Smith ED, Walsh-Burke K, Crusan C. Principles of training social workers in oncology." Chapter 92: *Principles of Training Social Workers in Oncology.* 2nd ed. New York: Oxford University Press; 2010: pp. 1061–1067

7. Blitz C. Meals on wheels, the effect of a home food-delivery service on cancer patients. https://clinicaltrials.gov/ct2/show/NCT02093312

Chapter 8

1. Scott WD. *Lung Cancer: A Guide to Diagnosis and Treatment.* Omaha, NE: Addicus Books, 2012.

2. Rabinoff M, Caskey N, Rissling A, Park C. Pharmacological and chemical effects of cigarette additives. *American Journal of Public Health.* 2007;97(11):1981–1991. doi:10.2105/AJPH.2005.078014

3. Baker F, Ainsworth SR, Dye JT, et al. Health risks associated with cigar smoking. *JAMA* 2000;284(6):735–740.

4. Hyland A, Piazza K, Hovey KM, et al. Associations between lifetime tobacco exposure with infertility and age at natural menopause: the Women's Health Initiative Observational Study [published online ahead of print December 14, 2015]. *Tobacco Control.* doi:10.1136/tobaccocontrol-2015-052510

5. Leonardi-Bee J, Britton J, Venn A. Secondhand smoke and adverse fetal outcomes in nonsmoking pregnant women: a meta-analysis. *Pediatrics.* 2011;127(4)734–741doi:10.1542/peds.2010-3041

6. Seddon JM, Willett WC, Speizer FE, Hankinson SE. A prospective study of cigarette smoking and age-related macular degeneration in women. *JAMA.* 1996;276(14):1141–1146. doi:10.1001/jama.1996.03540140029022

7. Peres J. No clear link between passive smoking and lung cancer [published online December 6, 2013]. *Journal of the National Cancer Institute.* doi:10.1093/jnci/djt365

8. Tavernise S. Secondhand smoke exposure drops, CDC reports. *New York Times.* February 3, 2013. http://www.nytimes.com/2015/02/04/health /for-americans-second-hand-smoke-exposure-cut-in-half-cdc-reports.html

9. Hang B, Sarker AH, Havel C, et al. Thirdhand smoke causes DNA damage in human cells. *Mutagenesis.* 2013;28(4):381–391. doi:10.1093/ mutage/get013

10. Benowitz NL, Hukkanen J, Jacob P. Nicotine chemistry, metabolism, kinetics and biomarkers. In *Handbook of Experimental Pharmacology.* 2009;(192):29–60. doi:10.1007/978-3-540-69248-5_2

11. Uhl GR, Drgon T, Johnson C, et al. Genome-wide association for smoking cessation success in a trial of precessation nicotine replacement. *Molecular Medicine.* 2010;16(11–12):513–526. doi:10.2119/molmed.2010 .00052.

12. Belsky DW, Moffitt TE, Baker TB, et al. Polygenic risk and the developmental progression to heavy, persistent smoking and nicotine dependence: evidence from a 4-decade longitudinal study. *JAMA Psychiatry.* 2013;70(5): 534–542. doi:10.1001/jamapsychiatry.2013.736

13. Park ER, Japuntich SJ, Rigotti NA, et al. A snapshot of smokers following lung and colorectal cancer diagnosis. *Cancer.* 2012;118(12):3153–3164. doi:10.1002/cncr.26545

14. Park ER, Japuntich SJ, Rigotti NA, et al. A snapshot of smokers following lung and colorectal cancer diagnosis. *Cancer.* 2012;118(12):3153–3164. doi:10.1002/cncr.26545

15. Farhat FS, Houhou W. Targeted therapies in non-small cell lung carcinoma: what have we achieved so far? *Therapeutic Advances in Medical Oncology.* 2013;5(4):249–270. doi:10.1177/1758834013492001

16. Johnson BE. Second lung cancers in patients after treatment for an initial lung cancer. *Journal of the National Cancer Institute.* 1998;90(18): 1335–1345 doi:10.1093/jnci/90.18.1335

17. Galanti LM. Tobacco smoking cessation management: integrating varenicline in current practice. *Vascular Health and Risk Management.* 2008;4(4):837–845.

18. Ogbru O. Nicotine polacrilex (Nicotine Gum, Nicorelief, Nicorette, Thrive). *MedicineNet.* http://www.medicinenet.com/nicotine_gum/article .htm

19. Shiffman S. Gradual smoking reduction using nicotine gum. *American Journal of Preventive Medicine.* 2008;36(2):96–014. doi: http://dx.doi.org /10.1016/j.amepre.2008.09.039

20. Foulds J. Nicotrol nasal spray: an effective treatment for the heavy smoker. Healthline Blogs. http://www.healthline.com/health-blogs/freedom-smoking/nicotrol-nasal-spray-effective-treatment-heavy-smoker

21. Ebbert JO, Hughes JR, West RJ, et al. Effect of varenicline on smoking cessation through smoking reduction: a randomized clinical trial. *JAMA.* 2015;313(7):687–694. doi: 10.1001/jama.2015.280

22. Wilkes S. The use of bupropion SR in cigarette smoking cessation. *International Journal of Chronic Obstructive Pulmonary Disease.* 2008; 3(1):45–53. PMCID: PMC2528204

23. Tombor I, Shahab L, Brown J, Notley C, West R. Does non-smoker identity following quitting predict long-term abstinence? Evidence from a population survey in England. *Addictive Behaviors.* 2015;45:99–103. doi:10.1016/j.addbeh.2015.01.026. *BMJ Open* 2016;6:6 e011045 doi:10.1136/bmjopen-2016-011045

Chapter 9

1. Kübler-Ross E. *On Death and Dying: What the Dying Have to Teach Doctors, Nurses, Clergy and Their Own Families* (reprint ed.). New York: Scribner, 2014.

2. Petticrew M, Bell R, Hunter D. Influence of psychological coping on survival and recurrence in people with cancer: systematic review. *BMJ.* 2002;325(7372):1066.

3. El-Hellani A, El-Hage R, Baalbaki R, et al. Free-base and protonated nicotine in electronic cigarette liquids and aerosols. *Chemical Research in Toxicology.* 2015;28(8):1532–1537. doi: 10.1021/acs.chemrestox.5b00107

4. National Institute of Mental Health. Depression. http://www.nimh.nih.gov/health/topics/depression/men-and-depression/signs-and-symptoms-of-depression/index.shtml

5. National Institute of Mental Health. Anxiety disorders. http://www.nimh.nih.gov/health/topics/anxiety-disorders/index.shtml

Glossary

Adjuvant therapy—Any therapy that starts after surgery.

Benign—Noncancerous (nonharmful) in effect.

Biomarkers—A distinctive substance that indicates a particular disease is present.

Bronchi—One of two passages within the trachea that allow air into the lungs.

Carcinogens—Substances that cause cancer.

Chemotherapy regimen—A combination of chemotherapy drugs.

DNA (deoxyribonucleic acid)—The molecule in every cell that controls how that cell grows and functions.

Fiducial marker—A small gold seed or platinum coil that is placed around a tumor to act as a radiological and mark.

Free radicals—Molecules formed in the body due to exposure to carcinogens. These damage cells and alter a cell's DNA.

Genetic fusion—A gene that is formed when the genetic material from two previously separate genes are mixed.

Genetic mutation—A change in the structure of a gene.

Hemoptysis—Coughing up of blood or blood-stained sputum.

Lymph nodes—The part of the lymph system responsible for filtering wastes out of the liquid that passes through the bloodstream.

Lymphatic system—The system responsible for transporting nutrients to the body's cells and carrying waste away from the cells.

Malignant—Uncontrollable or infectious disease.

Mesothelium—The lining that covers the body's internal organs and cavities.

Metastasis—Cancer that moves from its site of origination to another part of the body.

Molecular testing—Also called assays or profiles, molecular testing can help your treatment team identify specific biomarkers that are in a tumor.

Neoadjuvant therapy—Any therapy (chemotherapy or radiation) that starts before surgery.

Next-generation sequencing—A technique or method of accurately sequencing large amounts of DNA in a short period of time.

Pleura—The outer lining of the lungs.

Pleurodesis—A therapy offered to lung cancer patients to remove excess fluid (called pleural effusion) from the space between the lungs and chest wall.

Primary lung cancer—Lung cancer that starts in the lung.

Prophylactic cranial irradiation (PCI)—A kind of radiation treatment that may be used to kill cancer cells in the brain that may not be visible on X-rays or scans.

Radioactive isotope—An atom that emits radiation that can be seen by radiological equipment.

Secondary lung cancer—Cancer that forms in another part of the body and travels to the lung.

Thoracoscope—A camera on the end of flexible tubing that enables a doctor to look into the chest.

Trachea—Also known as the "windpipe"; a tube that connects the pharynx or larynx to the lungs, allowing the passage of air.

Tumor—A group of cells that stick together. Tumors can be benign (noncancerous) or malignant (cancerous).

Index

Note: *Italicized* page numbers indicate information found in tables.

About the Author

As a leading thoracic surgeon specializing in minimally invasive sur-gery, and a much sought-after authority on all things lung cancer, Dr. Eric R. Presser has successfully maintained his affiliations with traditional allopathic medicine while associating with and learning from a wide range of complementary practitioners. Since 1999, he has been an innovative doctor with a thriving career in both clinical and surgical settings. He is currently an attending thoracic surgeon at Premier Surgical Associates in Palm Springs, California, and an as-sociate professor at the University of California Riverside School of Medicine. After earning an undergraduate degree in microbiology and double minors in chemistry and gerontology at the University of Florida in Gainesville, he received a medical degree with honors from Ross University School of Medicine. Dr. Presser completed his surgi-cal internship and residency at St. Vincent Hospital and Medical Center in New York City, where he was appointed to the position of chief resident. In 2006, after spending a year in cardiothoracic train-ing at Louisiana State University in New Orleans, Dr. Presser went on to complete his fellowship in cardiothoracic surgery at the University of Texas Science Center in San Antonio. He also served as an associate professor of surgery at Hofstra North Shore-LIJ School of Medicine on Long Island.

Dr. Presser's contributions to the field of minimally invasive tho-racic surgery are considerable. In particular, his approach to com-mon medical scenarios involving lung masses, lung cancer, and pathology in the chest is widely viewed as "cutting edge," and he has pioneered new minimally invasive approaches for complex surgical problems that, in the past, have mandated days to weeks of hospitalization. As an example, he performs all major lung resections using the smallest incisions possible, including a single-incision VATS (video-assisted thoracic surgery) and even "awake" thoracoscopy for those patients too sick or afraid to undergo general anesthesia when needed.

Without a doubt, Dr. Presser's proudest accomplishments are those that eliminate the pain and discomfort associated with conventional surgery, allowing patients to return almost immediately to their normal routines, often feeling as though the surgery has not taken place. "My goal is to have my patients spend less time in the hospital and more time enjoying their lives," he says.

Dr. Presser has brought the same focus, determination, and insight to the treatment of lung cancer. He lectures widely, both on the benefits of screening for prevention and early detection of lung cancer and on mesothelioma, the rare but deadly asbestos-related cancer that frequently manifests on the thin protective tissues that cover the lungs.

Dr. Presser is also board certified in hyperbaric medicine and wound care, which extends the scope of his practice outside the operating room. As part of his continuing commitment to providing comprehensive lung cancer care, Dr. Presser works closely with hospice and home health agencies to make sure the emotional and spiritual needs of patients with life-limiting illnesses are met and that they are comfortable and well cared for after leaving the hospital.

As an innovator and inventor, Dr. Presser has consulted with leading medical equipment companies, including Covidien, Life Technologies, and Galen Technologies. Dr. Presser serves on the board of the Desert Cancer Foundation, an organization that provides funding for cancer patients who can't afford medical care. He is a member of the medical advisory boards of Gilda's Club, the American Association for Thoracic Surgery, and the Society of Thoracic Surgeons.

Dr. Presser maintains a demanding schedule, traveling frequently for work and speaking engagements and participating in a number of high-profile programs and seminars around the country. Brilliant and charismatic, yet incredibly down to earth and plainspoken, Dr. Presser is a tireless crusader for changing the dynamic of lung cancer treatment. Nothing will stop him. Dr. Presser knows he's on the right course, particularly as the facts and proof continue to mount in favor of a prevention model for lung cancer. Equally telling is the growing number of more "experienced" surgeons who are adopting Dr. Presser's techniques.

Originally from New York, Dr. Presser now resides in Rancho Mirage, California, with his wife and two young children.

"I'm committed to changing the way we treat lung cancer, one patient at a time."

—Dr. Presser

6/17 Ø (1/16)